Minimizing, Recognizing, and Managing Endoscopic Adverse Events

Editors

UZMA D. SIDDIQUI
CHRISTOPHER J. GOSTOUT

GASTROINTESTINAL ENDOSCOPY CLINICS OF NORTH AMERICA

www.giendo.theclinics.com

Consulting Editor
CHARLES J. LIGHTDALE

January 2015 • Volume 25 • Number 1

ELSEVIER

1600 John F. Kennedy Boulevard ● Suite 1800 ● Philadelphia, Pennsylvania, 19103-2899

http://www.theclinics.com

GASTROINTESTINAL ENDOSCOPY CLINICS OF NORTH AMERICA Volume 25, Number 1
January 2015 ISSN 1052-5157, ISBN-13: 978-0-323-34175-2

Editor: Kerry Holland
Developmental Editor: Donald Mumford

Gastrointestinal Endoscopy Clinics of North America (ISSN 1052-5157) is published quarterly by Elsevier Inc., 360 Park Avenue South, New York, NY 10010-1710. Months of issue are January, April, July, and October. Business and Editorial Offices: 1600 John F. Kennedy Blvd., Suite 1800, Philadelphia, PA, 19103-2899. Periodicals postage paid at New York, NY and additional mailing offices. Subscription prices are $335.00 per year for US individuals, $486.00 per year for US institutions, $175.00 per year for US students and residents, $370.00 per year for Canadian individuals, $576.00 per year for Canadian institutions, $465.00 per year for international individuals, $576.00 per year for international institutions, and $245.00 per year for Canadian and foreign students/residents. To receive student/resident rate, orders must be accompanied by name of affiliated institution, date of term, and the *signature* of program/residency coordinator on institution letterhead. Orders will be billed at individual rate until proof of status is received. Foreign air speed delivery is included in all *Clinics* subscription prices. All prices are subject to change without notice. **POSTMASTER:** Send address change to *Gastrointestinal Endoscopy Clinics of North America*, Elsevier Health Sciences Division, Subscription Customer Service, 3251 Riverport Lane, Maryland Heights, MO 63043. **Customer Service: 1-800-654-2452 (US). From outside the United States, call 1-314-447-8871. Fax: 1-314-447-8029. E-mail: JournalsCustomerService-usa@elsevier.com (for print support) or JournalsOnlineSupport-usa@elsevier.com (for online support).**

Reprints. For copies of 100 or more, of articles in this publication, please contact the Commercial Reprints Department, Elsevier Inc., 360 Park Avenue South, New York, NY 10010-1710. Tel. 212-633-3874; Fax: 212-633-3820; E-mail: reprints@elsevier.com.

Gastrointestinal Endoscopy Clinics of North America is covered in *Excerpta Medica, MEDLINE/PubMed (Index Medicus), and MEDLINE/MEDLARS.*

Contributors

CONSULTING EDITOR

CHARLES J. LIGHTDALE, MD
Professor of Medicine, Division of Digestive and Liver Diseases, Columbia University Medical Center, New York, New York

EDITORS

UZMA D. SIDDIQUI, MD
Associate Professor of Medicine, University of Chicago Medicine, Center for Endoscopic Research and Therapeutics (CERT), Chicago, Illinois

CHRISTOPHER J. GOSTOUT, MD
Professor of Medicine, Division of Gastroenterology and Hepatology Mayo Clinic, Rochester, Minnesota

AUTHORS

DOUGLAS G. ADLER, MD, FACG, AGAF, FASGE
Associate Professor of Medicine; Director of Therapeutic Endoscopy; Director, GI Fellowship Program, Division of Gastroenterology and Hepatology, Department of Internal Medicine, University of Utah School of Medicine, Huntsman Cancer Center, Salt Lake City, Utah

CHRISTINE BOUMITRI, MD
Resident, Department of Medicine, Staten Island University Hospital, Staten Island, New York

DISAYA CHAVALITDHAMRONG, MD
Division of Gastroenterology, Hepatology and Nutrition, Department of Internal Medicine, University of Florida, Gainesville, Florida

PETER V. DRAGANOV, MD
Professor of Medicine; Division of Gastroenterology, Hepatology and Nutrition, Department of Internal Medicine, University of Florida, Gainesville, Florida

DAVID FRIEDEL, MD
Department of Gastroenterology, Hepatology and Nutrition, Winthrop University Hospital, Mineola, New York

ANDRES GELRUD, MD, MMSc
Associate Professor of Medicine, Division of Gastroenterology, Center for Endoscopic Research and Therapeutics (CERT), University of Chicago Medical Center, Chicago, Illinois

PRIYA A. JAMIDAR, MD, FACG, FASGE
Section of Digestive Diseases, Department of Internal Medicine, Yale University School of Medicine, New Haven, Connecticut

MICHEL KAHALEH, MD, FASGE
Professor of Medicine, Chief of Endoscopy, Division of Gastroenterology and Hepatology, Weill Cornell Medical College, New York, New York

NIKHIL A. KUMTA, MD
Fellow, Division of Gastroenterology and Hepatology, Weill Cornell Medical College, New York, New York

RANI MODAYIL, MD
Department of Gastroenterology, Hepatology and Nutrition, Winthrop University Hospital, Mineola, New York

MILAN PATEL, MD
Fellow, Division of Gastroenterology, Robert Wood Johnson Medical School, Mount Laurel, New Jersey

NAYANTARA COELHO PRABHU, MBBS
Assistant Professor, Division of Gastroenterology and Hepatology, Mayo Clinic, Rochester, Minnesota

JASON N. ROGART, MD, FASGE
Director of Interventional Gastroenterology and Therapeutic Endoscopy, Capital Health Center for Digestive Health, Pennington, New Jersey

TARUN RUSTAGI, MD
Section of Digestive Diseases, Department of Internal Medicine, Yale University School of Medicine, New Haven, Connecticut

AMRITA SETHI, MD
Assistant Professor of Medicine, Division of Digestive and Liver Diseases, Columbia University, New York, New York

AJAYPAL SINGH, MD
Division of Gastroenterology, Center for Endoscopic Research and Therapeutics (CERT), University of Chicago Medical Center, Chicago, Illinois

STAVROS N. STAVROPOULOS, MD
Department of Gastroenterology, Hepatology and Nutrition, Winthrop University Hospital, Mineola, New York

JOHN J. VARGO II, MD, MPH, AGAF, FACG, FASGE, FACP
Pier C. and Renee A. Borra Family Endowed Chair in Gastroenterology and Hepatology; Chair, Department of Gastroenterology and Hepatology; Vice Chair, Digestive Disease Institute, Cleveland Clinic, Cleveland, Ohio

LOUIS M. WONG KEE SONG, MD
Associate Professor of Medicine, Division of Gastroenterology and Hepatology, Mayo Clinic, Rochester, Minnesota

Contents

> Endoscopy constitutes a wide range of procedures with many indications. ophagogastroduodenoscopy, colonoscopy, endoscopic retrograde chol-angiopancreatography, endoscopic ultrasonography, and enteroscopy comprise the most commonly performed procedures. These examinations all carry risk to the patient, and incumbent in this is some legal risk with regard to how the procedure is conducted, decisions made based on the intraprocedure findings, and the postprocedure results, in addition to events that occur following the procedure. This article provides an over-view of consent and complications of endoscopy.

> Acute endoscopic perforations of the foregut and colon are rare but can have devastating consequences. There are several principles and prac-tices that can lower the risk of perforation and guide the endoscopist in early assessment when they do occur. Mastery of these principles will lead to overall improved patient outcomes.

> Luminal perforation after endoscopy is a dreaded complication that is associated with significant morbidity and mortality, longer and more costly hospitalization, and the specter of potential future litigation. The manage-ment of such perforations requires a multidisciplinary approach. Until recently, surgery was required. However, nowadays the endoscopist has a burgeoning armamentarium of devices and techniques that may obviate surgery. This article discusses the approach to endoscopic perforations in the esophagus and stomach.

> Early recognition of perforations arising from endoscopy is essential. In some cases the perforation can be viewed clearly during the procedure,

and immediate action should be taken to repair the defect endoscopically if feasible. If perforation is unclear, imaging can be used to confirm the diagnosis. Surgical intervention is not always necessary; however, a surgical consultation for backup is essential. Selective cases can be managed conservatively or endoscopically with successful outcomes. Early recognition and intervention, input from specialist colleagues, and communication with the patient and family are keys to successfully managing the event.

Amrita Sethi and Louis M. Wong Kee Song

 Videos demonstrating the prevention and management of adverse events associated with polypectomy and endoscopic mucosal resection of colonic lesions accompany this article

Colonoscopy is a commonly performed procedure. The rate of adverse events is 2.8 per 1000 screening colonoscopies. These adverse events include cardiovascular and pulmonary events, abdominal pain, hemorrhage, perforation, postpolypectomy syndrome, infection, and death. Serious adverse events, such as hemorrhage and perforation, occur most frequently when colonoscopy is performed with polypectomy. This article highlights the prevention and management of adverse events associated with polypectomy and endoscopic mucosal resection of colonic lesions.

Ajaypal Singh and Andres Gelrud

Placement of percutaneous endoscopic gastrostomy or jejunostomy is a safe procedure with low periprocedural mortality, but overall mortality rates are high because of underlying disease conditions. These procedures are also associated with postprocedure complications. The clinically significant adverse events related to the procedures include infection (at tube site and peritonitis), bleeding, and aspiration. More rare associated events include buried bumpers, injury to adjacent viscera with subsequent fistula formation, and tumor seeding. There is a lack of guidelines about these procedures other than those concerning the use of antibiotics and the management of antithrombotics and anticoagulation before the procedure.

Disaya Chavalitdhamrong, Douglas G. Adler, and Peter V. Draganov

Deep small bowel enteroscopy is a safe procedure that has revolutionized the strategy for diagnosis and treatment of small bowel diseases. However, enteroscopy-associated adverse events are more common compared with standard endoscopy. Prevention, early detection, and effective intervention are crucial in reducing the adverse event severity and improving outcomes. In this article, how to safely perform enteroscopy, avoid adverse events, detect adverse events early, and accomplish effective treatments are discussed. This knowledge can serve as a continuing quality improvement process to reduce the risk of future adverse events and improve the overall quality of endoscopy.

Endoscopic retrograde cholangiopancreatography (ERCP) represents a monumental advance in the management of patients with pancreaticobiliary diseases, but is a complex and technically demanding procedure with the highest inherent risk of adverse events of all routine endoscopic procedures. Overall adverse event rates for ERCP are typically reported as 5–10%. The most commonly reported adverse events include post-ERCP pancreatitis, bleeding, perforation, infection (cholangitis), and cardiopulomary or "sedation related" events. This article evaluates patient-related and procedure-related risk factors for ERCP-related adverse events, and discusses strategies for the prevention, diagnosis and management of these events.

Post–endoscopic retrograde cholangiopancreatography pancreatitis (PEP) is the most common complication of endoscopic retrograde cholangiopancreatography (ERCP), and not uncommonly is the reason behind ERCP-related lawsuits. Patients at high risk for PEP include young women with abdominal pain, normal liver tests, and unremarkable imaging. Procedure-related factors include traumatic and persistent cannulation attempts, multiple injections of the pancreatic duct, pancreatic sphincterotomy, and, possibly, use of precut sphincterotomy. Aggressive hydration, use of rectal indomethacin, and prophylactic pancreatic stenting can diminish the risk (and likely severity) of PEP. Though hugely beneficial, these measures do not supersede careful patient selection and technique.

 Videos demonstrating endoscopic hemostasis accompany this article

Acute gastrointestinal bleeding is a common cause for hospitalization. Endoscopic hemostasis plays a central role in the management of lesions with active bleeding or high-risk stigmata for rebleeding. The efficacy and safety of endoscopic hemostasis rely on the identification of lesions suitable for endoscopic therapy, selection of the appropriate hemostatic devices, attention to technique, and prompt recognition and management of procedure-related adverse events. In this article, practical applications of hemostatic devices and pitfalls related to endoscopic hemostasis are discussed.

Defining the risk of procedural sedation for gastrointestinal endoscopic procedures remains a vexing challenge. The definitions as to what constitutes a cardiopulmonary unplanned event are beginning to take focus but the existing literature is an amalgam of various definitions and subjective outcomes, providing a challenge to patient, practitioner, and researcher. Gastrointestinal endoscopy when undertaken by trained personnel after the appropriate preprocedural evaluation and in the right setting is a safe experience. However, significant challenges exist in further quantifying the sedation risks to patients, optimizing physiologic monitoring, and sublimating the pharmacoeconomic and regulatory embroglios that limit the scope of practice and the quality of services delivered to patients.

Increasingly invasive therapeutic endoscopic and laparoscopic procedures have resulted in endoscopists more frequently encountering complications including perforations, fistulas, and anastomotic leakages, for which nonsurgical closure is desired. Devices and techniques are available and in development for endoscopic closure of gastrointestinal wall defects. Currently available devices with excellent clinical success rates include the over-the-scope clip and an endoscopic suturing system. Another device, the cardiac septal defect occluder, has been adapted for use in the gastrointestinal tract. Extensive endoscopic knowledge, a highly trained endoscopy team, and the availability of devices and equipment are required to effectively manage complications endoscopically.

GASTROINTESTINAL ENDOSCOPY CLINICS OF NORTH AMERICA

ISSUE OF RELATED INTEREST

Gastroenterology Clinics of North America, March 2014, (Vol 43, No. 1)
Gastroesophageal Reflux Disease
Joel Richter, *Editor*

Foreword

Comprehensive Review of Adverse Events Associated with GI Endoscopy

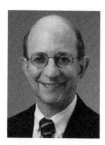

Charles J. Lightdale, MD
Consulting Editor

Complications directly related to gastrointestinal endoscopy are infrequent, but must be discussed with patients before endoscopy, diagnosed during or as soon as possible after endoscopy, and treated appropriately. One of my old teachers used to call endoscopic adverse events: "the price of doing business." As GI endoscopy procedures have evolved from largely diagnostic to more interventional, often with therapeutic intent, "the price" has gone up. The most striking recent change is the ability to manage many complications, such as bleeding or perforation, with new endoscopic tools that have been utilized in interventional procedures or that have been designed with the treatment of specific adverse events in mind.

The editors for this issue of the *Gastrointestinal Endoscopy Clinics of North America* on the subject of "Minimizing, Recognizing, and Managing Endoscopic Adverse Events," Dr Uzma Siddiqui and Dr Christopher J. Gostout have taken a comprehensive approach to this task. From completing and documenting informed consent, to minimizing complications, and recognizing and successfully managing them when they occur, every endoscopic procedure from common to highly interventional is discussed by a remarkably qualified and experienced group of specialists. This is a clear-eyed, nothing-held-back review of endoscopic complications that should be studied in

Gastrointest Endoscopy Clin N Am 25 (2015) xi–xii
http://dx.doi.org/10.1016/j.giec.2014.10.002
1052-5157/15/$ – see front matter © 2015 Elsevier Inc. All rights reserved.

detail by all gastrointestinal endoscopists and should be available in every setting where GI endoscopy is performed.

Charles J. Lightdale, MD
Professor of Medicine
Division of Digestive and Liver Diseases
Columbia University Medical Center
161 Fort Washington Avenue, Room 812
New York, NY 10032, USA

E-mail address:
CJL18@columbia.edu

Preface

Minimizing, Recognizing, and Managing Endoscopic Adverse Events

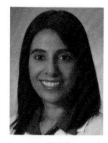 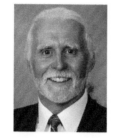

Uzma D. Siddiqui, MD   Christopher J. Gostout, MD
Editors

This issue of *Gastrointestinal Endoscopy Clinics of North America* entitled, "Minimizing, Recognizing, and Managing Endoscopic Adverse Events," is a comprehensive review of possible undesirable outcomes related to all types of endoscopic procedures. As the number of endoscopic procedures performed continues to increase, so does the potential for adverse events (AE). Previous articles and endoscopy courses may have addressed a specific type of AE related to one or two endoscopic procedures; however, this issue explores the full range of endoscopic AE.

The following articles discuss not only AE themselves but also the keys to improving patient care through proper informed consent, adequate preparation for a procedure, prompt recognition when an AE has happened, and the use of devices to assist with endoscopic management when appropriate. The authors are all expert endoscopists from around the country, whose knowledge of this topic should be far ranging and who are experienced in use of the latest technology to aid in the management of AE.

The text should serve as a valuable resource for anyone performing or assisting with endoscopic procedures, including gastroenterologists, fellows, nurses, and technicians. Being part of an endoscopy team means being prepared for the unexpected. This issue will help achieve that goal.

Uzma D. Siddiqui, MD
Associate Professor of Medicine
University of Chicago Medicine
Center for Endoscopic Research and Therapeutics (CERT)
5700 S. Maryland Avenue, MC 8043
Chicago, IL 60637

Gastrointest Endoscopy Clin N Am 25 (2015) xiii–xiv
http://dx.doi.org/10.1016/j.giec.2014.10.001
1052-5157/15/$ – see front matter © 2015 Elsevier Inc. All rights reserved.

Christopher J. Gostout, MD
Professor of Medicine
Division of Gastroenterology and Hepatology Mayo Clinic
200 1st ST SW, Rochester, MN 55905

E-mail addresses:
usiddiqui@bsd.uchicago.edu (U.D. Siddiqui)
gostout.christopher@mayo.edu (C.J. Gostout)

Consent, Common Adverse Events, and Post–Adverse Event Actions in Endoscopy

Douglas G. Adler, MD

KEYWORDS

- Adverse events • Medicolegal • Open-access endoscopy • Postprocedural care

KEY POINTS

- Despite being exceptionally safe overall, modern endoscopy carries significant risks of adverse events.
- Most adverse events can be treated endoscopically, but in rare cases surgery or other interventions will be needed.
- A proper consent and clear communication of the risks, benefits, and alternatives to a procedure are helpful in setting realistic expectations of what to expect both during and after a procedure.
- Establishing a good doctor-patient relationship before a procedure can alleviate some of the stress induced once an endoscopic adverse event occurs, and only helps to provide improved clinical care for the patient.

INTRODUCTION

Endoscopy constitutes a wide range of procedures with many indications. Esophago-gastroduodenoscopy, colonoscopy, endoscopic retrograde cholangiopancreatography (ERCP), endoscopic ultrasonography (EUS), and enteroscopy comprise the most commonly performed procedures. These examinations all carry risk to the patient, and incumbent in this is some legal risk with regard to how the procedure is conducted, decisions made based on the intraprocedure findings, and the postproce-dure results, in addition to events that occur following the procedure. This article provides an overview of consent and complications of endoscopy.

PATIENT SELECTION

Patient selection for endoscopy is often straightforward but always has some medi-colegal implications. If the patient is known to you, has been seen in your clinic previ-ously, and you have reviewed their history, examined the patient, and so forth, you have most likely appropriately recommended a procedure based on their history, problem, and current and future needs.

GI Fellowship Program, Gastroenterology and Hepatology, University of Utah School of Medicine, Huntsman Cancer Center, 30N 1900E 4R118, Salt Lake City, UT 84312, USA
E-mail address: douglas.adler@hsc.utah.edu

Gastrointest Endoscopy Clin N Am 25 (2015) 1–8
http://dx.doi.org/10.1016/j.giec.2014.09.001
1052-5157/15/$ – see front matter © 2015 Elsevier Inc. All rights reserved.

Open-access endoscopy is completely within the standard of care. Open-access endoscopy, which is widely performed, presents challenges, as the history and physical examination are performed in the immediate preprocedure setting, and in most cases these can be resolved. When practicing open-access endoscopy, the following should be considered:

- Is the patient an appropriate candidate for the intended procedure?
- Does the patient understand the nature of the proposed procedure?
- Does the patient understand the risks of the proposed procedure, and the consequences of an adverse event?
- Does the patient have comorbid illnesses that would make the intended procedure unwise?
- Does the patient understand that they may need multiple procedures going forward to accomplish the endoscopic goals?
- Does the patient understand that surgery may be required if endoscopic approaches fail?
- Does the patient have adequate time to have any procedure-related questions asked and answered?

INFORMED CONSENT

A perfect informed consent does not exist, and there can always be some disagreement on what constitutes a well-crafted informed consent, especially after an adverse event. As has been said many times, so much so that it is almost a mantra, informed consent is a process and not simply a piece of paper. Many physicians delegate the process of obtaining the actual informed consent to nonphysicians (nurses, medical assistants, medical students, and so forth). Although not required, a good rule of thumb is that one of the physicians who will be performing the intended procedure should be the one to obtain the informed consent from the patient if at all possible. As such, it is completely acceptable for either the attending physician or a gastrointestinal (GI) fellow to obtain consent on a procedure performed jointly by an attending physician and a fellow. Consent should ideally give the patient adequate time to ask any and all relevant questions. Many patients would like to have family present at the time of consent, and if this is the case they should also have the opportunity to ask questions. Informed consent for endoscopy should include a review of the risks, benefits, alternatives to the procedure, and nature of the procedure itself, in addition to the following potential complications:

- Bleeding
- Allergic/cardiac/respiratory reaction
- Bowel perforation with the possible need for emergency surgery
- Pancreatitis for patients undergoing ERCP or EUS with pancreatic fine-needle aspiration (which can be severe)
- Infection
- Missed lesions (usually in the case of colonoscopy)

OVERVIEW OF KEY ADVERSE EVENTS

This section is a brief introduction to a few of the most commonly encountered adverse events related to endoscopy. More detailed reviews can be found elsewhere in this issue.

Post–Endoscopic Retrograde Cholangiopancreatography Pancreatitis

Post-ERCP pancreatitis (PEP) remains the most common and most feared adverse outcome in the realm of therapeutic endoscopy. The reported incidence of PEP for diagnostic and therapeutic ERCP is 0.4% to 1.5% and 1.6% to 5.4%, respectively. High-risk cohorts (patients with sphincter of Oddi dysfunction [SOD] undergoing ERCP) have a much higher rate of PEP.[1]

Patient-related factors have been extensively evaluated, and include suspected or known SOD (raising the rate to 10%–30%[2–5]) as well as prior PEP (18%–26%)[3,4,6] A normal serum bilirubin also carries an increased risk of PEP.[3,7,8] Previous pancreatitis, even when not due to an ERCP, also increases the risk of PEP.[5,7]

Young patient age (usually considered <30 years) is associated with an increased risk of PEP.[3,5] Female gender is a well-established risk factor for PEP, with a relative risk of 2.23.[3,5,7,8] Current and former alcohol users/abusers, along with former smokers, have a 2- to 3-fold risk for PEP.[9] The presence of pancreas divisum increases the risk of PEP to 8.2% when dorsal pancreatic duct cannulation is attempted (even if not successful).[7] Multiple high-risk factors seem to have a cumulative increase in the risk of developing PEP (ie, a young woman with presumed SOD and normal serum bilirubin).[3]

Conversely, there are a few patient-related or disease-related factors that seem to impart a lower rate of PEP. For example, elderly patients experience a lower rate of PEP when compared with younger patients, and these patients tolerate ERCP well overall.[8] A study looking at combined ERCP and EUS in elderly patients showed that this approach was considered safe and effective, even in very elderly patients, and even when taking into account the increased length of the procedure and the need for deep sedation/general anesthesia.[10] Patients with pancreatic solid tumors (most commonly pancreatic adenocarcinoma of the head) are at decreased risk for PEP when undergoing purely biliary procedures, owing to chronic obstruction of the pancreatic duct along with atrophy of the upstream pancreatic parenchyma.[11]

With regard to procedure-related factors, several are known to increase the risk of PEP. The so-called difficult cannulation is a nonspecific term that is used to refer to a failure to obtain biliary access in a rapid or straightforward manner, and typically implies multiple and/or prolonged attempts at achieving deep biliary cannulation (whether or not cannulation was actually achieved). The term often implies that a combination of factors may have occurred during an attempt at cannulation, including the possibilities of associated mucosal trauma to the ampulla from repeated cannulation attempts, use of the needle-knife sphincterotomy technique, and/or multiple undesired pancreatic duct injections. Patients with a difficult cannulation are at an elevated risk of developing PEP.[3,4,6]

Needle-knife sphincterotomy is an established independent risk factor for PEP.[5] Some of the risk related to needle-knife sphincterotomy seems to be because a large number of cannulation attempts performed before the technique is used in most cases, arguing for the acceptability of early needle-knife attempts if standard approaches fail. Some of the risk is also due to the nature of the needle-knife sphincterotomy itself (ie, cautery to access the bile or pancreatic duct without a guide wire to ensure proper access and orientation when making the sphincterotomy). A retrospective study by Testoni and colleagues[12] showed that the rate of PEP is lower when needle-knife sphincterotomy was initiated after fewer than 10 cannulation attempts, which many would consider a very early transition to this technique (ie, most physicians would likely continue to attempt to achieve cannulation by standard techniques after 10 failed attempts). A 2010 meta-analysis by Cennamo and colleagues[13] demonstrated PEP in 2.5% of patients randomized to early needle-knife sphincterotomy, compared with 5.3% of patients undergoing persistent cannulation attempts before needle-knife sphincterotomy, also arguing that earlier application of this technique may be warranted over continued attempts at cannulation with standard devices, although this conclusion has not been embraced by the wider GI community.

Endoscopic papillary balloon dilation (EPBD) without prior biliary sphincterotomy has been associated with a high rate of PEP and adverse outcomes in Western patients, although it is much more commonly performed in Asia, most notably Japan. In a well-publicized, randomized controlled trial, EPBD without sphincterotomy was associated with a significantly increased risk of PEP, and the study included 2 deaths from pancreatitis occurring in patients who underwent EPBD without biliary sphincterotomy.[14] PEP is widely known to be associated with repeated pancreatic duct injections.[4]

Indomethacin as a prophylactic agent is widely being used in patients undergoing ERCP, based on a recent *New England Journal of Medicine* study showing a reduced incidence of PEP in those receiving 1 dose of rectal indomethacin at the conclusion of their ERCP. In this study, most patients (82%) were considered at high risk for PEP because they had suspected SOD. Therefore, the use of indomethacin in all patients undergoing ERCP as opposed to only selected high-risk patients is currently under debate.[15] However, given the ease and safety of a single dose regimen and its low cost, the routine use of rectal indomethacin as a PEP-preventive measure is gaining popularity.

Perforation

Risk factors that increase the potential for perforation to occur during endoscopy have been identified, and physicians should be aware of the more common ones. Endoscopic dilation of strictures (especially in patients with inflammatory bowel disease, most notably Crohn disease) or large-caliber dilation in achalasia are considered to be higher-risk procedures with regard to perforation. Furthermore, the performance of endoscopic mucosal resection or endoscopic submucosal dissection should also be considered a relatively high-risk procedure with regard to transluminal perforation in comparison with standard endoscopy.[16] Chronic steroid use can also increase the risk of perforation during any endoscopic procedure.

In patients undergoing ERCP, perforation is most likely to occur during sphincterotomy, but can also occur during intubation of the patient at the esophagus, stomach, or duodenum. Perforations may be more common in patients with postsurgical anatomy. Most sphincterotomy-related perforations are retroperitoneal and, if recognized, can often be managed conservatively with nil by mouth status, antibiotics, and close monitoring.[17] It should be mentioned that small retroperitoneal perforations might be difficult to identify clinically during ERCP.

Small bowel enteroscopy, once an uncommon procedure performed mostly at tertiary referral centers, is now in widespread use in both academic and community practices, as a result of the dissemination of several new endoscopic techniques (eg, single-balloon enteroscopy, double-balloon enteroscopy, spiral enteroscopy) that are now available to practitioners to allow them access to the entire small bowel, in either an anterograde or retrograde fashion. Perforations during these types of enteroscopy procedures are more likely to occur during interventions such as the treatment of bleeding, strictures, and when attempting to remove large polyps, although perforations can occur during advancement or removal of the endoscope, especially in patients with postsurgical anatomy.[18,19]

In patients with inflammatory bowel disease, patient-related risk factors associated with higher rates of perforation include severe/active inflammatory bowel disease, active or long-term corticosteroid use, female sex, older age, and the performance of endoscopic dilations (se earlier discussion).[20,21]

Elderly patients (variously defined as >60, 65, or 70 years) have been noted to have an increased risk of perforation, as have patients with multiple comorbidities.[22] Elderly patients can also have an increased risk of cardiopulmonary complications, and these must be addressed before the procedure, especially when planning for the appropriate type of anesthesia to administer and the need for additional anesthesia support. Other factors that increase the risk of perforation include extensive diverticular disease, multiple abdominal or pelvic surgeries (which can cause fixation of the colon resulting from adhesions), and bowel obstruction.[23,24]

Historically, transmural perforation of the bowel at almost any location mandated surgery to repair, but this dogma is rapidly changing. The increasing use of endoscopic clipping has allowed many of these perforations to be directly closed endoscopically. These clips work best if the perforation is focal, well visualized, and if there has been a paucity of or no soiling of the abdomen with enteric contents.[25,26] Through-the-scope or over-the-scope clips are widely available and are highly effective for treating small or localized perforations, but may fail to close perforations with a large transmural defect. Endoscopic suturing devices are also available.[27,28] Large perforations, perforations that cannot be seen well, or patients who have soiling of the abdomen with copious amounts of enteric contents will likely need surgery to repair these defects.

Bleeding

Bleeding, especially significant bleeding requiring transfusion or other interventions, is a rare event in modern endoscopy. Nonetheless, at some point all endoscopists are likely to cause a clinically significant bleed.

Postpolypectomy bleeding

Postpolypectomy bleeding represents a common adverse event, and all polypectomies place patients at some risk of bleeding. Risk factors for bleeding during a procedure include large polyps (>1 cm), polyps with thick stalks, renal disease (implying platelet dysfunction), anticoagulants, and cutting of the polyp by mistake before appropriate electrocautery is applied. Bleeding may be more common in patients undergoing piecemeal resection of large polyps.[29] Postpolypectomy bleeding can be immediate or delayed (ie, up to 1 week following a polypectomy) in development. Prophylactic clipping of polypectomy sites is widely used if the endoscopist is concerned about postpolypectomy bleeding, although this does increase the overall cost of the procedure.

Most delayed bleeding following colonoscopy can be managed endoscopically. Many postpolypectomy bleeding episodes stop by the time a repeat colonoscopy can be performed. Delayed bleeding following polypectomy is almost certainly underreported. Bleeding that is obscure, microscopic, and/or self-limited may go unnoticed by the patient.

Sphincterotomy-related bleeding

Sphincterotomy-related bleeding can be acute and visualized directly during the index ERCP, or can present in a delayed manner, often occurring several days following a procedure. Self-limited bleeding following sphincterotomy is often of no clinical concern. Major bleeds can occur in cirrhotic patients, patients requiring anticoagulation or antiplatelet medications, or in those for whom an intraduodenal blood vessel of significant size is transected during sphincterotomy. Major risk factors for postsphincterotomy bleeding include a significantly elevated prothrombin time (>2× upper limit of normal), hemodialysis (usually because of platelet dysfunction from underlying uremia), and significant bleeding at the time of the sphincterotomy (even if it stops spontaneously).[30] A meta-analysis by Verma and colleagues[31] studying sphincterotomy-related adverse events using pure versus mixed electrosurgical current demonstrated that pure cutting current was associated with more episodes of bleeding, although most were mild. At present, blended current or generators that alternate current waveforms are almost universally in use. Sphincterotomy-related bleeding can be treated by a variety of means, including direct endoscopic tamponade (often via the use of a biliary occlusion balloon), endoscopic clips, thermal therapy, and injection therapy. Endoscopic clips have a high failure rate when used through a duodenoscope, owing to angulation and bending of the clipping device at the elevator. Surgery or interventional radiology approaches may be needed for intractable bleeds.

POST–ADVERSE EVENT BEHAVIOR

Once an adverse event has occurred, the nature of the event should be disclosed to the patient and/or their family or legal representative as soon as possible. In some cases the adverse event will not be recognized immediately or may develop after the procedure has been completed and the patient has been discharged. This can present a difficulty for physicians if they are not aware an adverse event has occurred. In addition, the proposed steps to treat the event should also be disclosed so that questions and concerns can be voiced. These communications should be documented to reflect the ongoing doctor-patient interaction. Patients may be calm and accepting of the news of an adverse event, or be upset, tearful, and angry. Patients and their families should be able to reach the treating physicians for further information and for an ongoing plan of care.

In general, it seems more interaction is better than less interaction. If the patient must be handed off to another service (ie, surgery), the endoscopist should still be involved as much as possible in the care of the patient. In some cases, the endoscopist will have little to add if the required intervention is outside of their realm but, if possible, it is always worthwhile to maintain good contact with the patient and to document such encounters in the medical record.

Sometimes the patient may be treated for an adverse event at another hospital. It may be impossible for the initial physician to visit the patient in this situation. If possible, active lines of communication between the patient, family, and new treating physicians should be maintained to facilitate optimal outcomes.

SUMMARY

Despite being exceptionally safe overall, modern endoscopy carries significant risks of adverse events. Most adverse events can be treated endoscopically, but in rare cases surgery or other interventions will be needed. A proper consent and clear communication of the risks, benefits, and alternatives to a procedure are extremely helpful in setting realistic expectations of what to expect both during and after a procedure. Establishing a good doctor-patient relationship before a procedure can alleviate some of the stress induced once an endoscopic adverse event occurs, and can only help to provide improved clinical care for the patient.

REFERENCES

1. Arata S, Takada T, Hirata K, et al. Post-ERCP pancreatitis. J Hepatobiliary Pancreat Sci 2010;17(1):70–8.
2. Freeman ML, DiSario JA, Nelson DB, et al. Risk factors for post-ERCP pancreatitis: a prospective, multicenter study. Gastrointest Endosc 2001;54:425–34.

3. Freeman ML, Nelson DB, Sherman S, et al. Complications of endoscopic biliary sphincterotomy. N Engl J Med 1996;335:909–18.
4. Masci E, Toti G, Mariani A, et al. Complications of diagnostic and therapeutic ERCP: a prospective multicenter study. Am J Gastroenterol 2001;96:417–23.
5. Testoni PA, Mariani A, Giussani A, et al, SEIFRED Group. Risk factors for post-ERCP pancreatitis in high- and low-volume centers and among expert and non-expert operators: a prospective multicenter study. Am J Gastroenterol 2010;105(8):1753–61.
6. Vandervoort J, Soetikno RM, Tham TC, et al. Risk factors for complications after performance of ERCP. Gastrointest Endosc 2002;56:652–6.
7. Moffatt DC, Coté GA, Avula H, et al. Risk factors for ERCP-related complications in patients with pancreas divisum: a retrospective study. Gastrointest Endosc 2011;73(5):963–70.
8. Lukens FJ, Howell DA, Upender S, et al. ERCP in the very elderly: outcomes among patients older than eighty. Dig Dis Sci 2010;55(3):847–51.
9. Debenedet AT, Raghunathan TE, Wing JJ, et al. Alcohol use and cigarette smoking as risk factors for post-endoscopic retrograde cholangiopancreatography pancreatitis. Clin Gastroenterol Hepatol 2009;7:353–8.e4.
10. Iles-Shih L, Hilden K, Adler DG. Combined ERCP and EUS in one session is safe in elderly patients when compared to non-elderly patients: outcomes in 206 combined procedures. Dig Dis Sci 2012;57(7):1949–53. http://dx.doi.org/10.1007/s10620-012-2135-2.
11. Banerjee N, Hilden K, Baron TH, et al. Endoscopic biliary sphincterotomy is not required for transpapillary SEMS placement for biliary obstruction. Dig Dis Sci 2011;56(2):591–5.
12. Testoni PA, Giussani A, Vailati C, et al. Precut sphincterotomy, repeated cannulation and post-ERCP pancreatitis in patients with bile duct stone disease. Dig Liver Dis 2011;43(10):792–6.
13. Cennamo V, Fuccio L, Zagari RM, et al. Can early precut implementation reduce endoscopic retrograde cholangiopancreatography-related complication risk? Meta-analysis of randomized controlled trials. Endoscopy 2010;42(5):381–8.
14. Disario JA, Freeman ML, Bjorkman DJ, et al. Endoscopic balloon dilation compared with sphincterotomy for extraction of bile duct stones. Gastroenterology 2004;127(5):1291–9.
15. Elmunzer BJ, Scheiman JM, Lehman GA, et al, U.S. Cooperative for Outcomes Research in Endoscopy (USCORE). A randomized trial of rectal indomethacin to prevent post-ERCP pancreatitis. N Engl J Med 2012;366(15):1414–22. http://dx.doi.org/10.1056/NEJMoa1111103.
16. Park YM, Cho E, Kang HY, et al. The effectiveness and safety of endoscopic submucosal dissection compared with endoscopic mucosal resection for early gastric cancer: a systematic review and meta analysis. Surg Endosc 2011;25(8):2666–77.
17. Avgerinos DV, Llaguna OH, Lo AY, et al. Management of endoscopic retrograde cholangiopancreatography: related duodenal perforations. Surg Endosc 2009;23(4):833–8.
18. May A, Nachbar L, Pohl J, et al. Endoscopic interventions in the small bowel using double balloon enteroscopy: feasibility and limitations. Am J Gastroenterol 2007;102:527–35.
19. Aktas H, de Ridder L, Haringsma J, et al. Complications of single-balloon enteroscopy: a prospective evaluation of 166 procedures. Endoscopy 2010;42:365–8.

20. Navaneethan U, Parasa S, Venkatesh PG, et al. Prevalence and risk factors for colonic perforation during colonoscopy in hospitalized inflammatory bowel disease patients. J Crohns Colitis 2011;5(3):189–95.
21. Navaneethan U, Kochhar G, Phull H, et al. Severe disease on endoscopy and steroid use increase the risk for bowel perforation during colonoscopy in inflammatory bowel disease patients. J Crohns Colitis 2012;6(4):470–5.
22. Arora G, Mannalithara A, Singh G, et al. Risk of perforation from a colonoscopy in adults: a large population-based study. Gastrointest Endosc 2009;69:654–64.
23. Gatto NM, Frucht H, Sundararajan V, et al. Risk of perforation after colonoscopy and sigmoidoscopy: a population-based study. J Natl Cancer Inst 2003;95: 230–6.
24. Korman LY, Overholt BF, Box T, et al. Perforation during colonoscopy in endoscopic ambulatory surgical centers. Gastrointest Endosc 2003;58:554–7.
25. Mönkemüller K, Peter S, Toshniwal J, et al. Multipurpose use of the 'bear claw' (over-the-scope-clip system) to treat endoluminal gastrointestinal disorders. Dig Endosc 2014;26(3):350–7. http://dx.doi.org/10.1111/den.12145.
26. Nishiyama N, Mori H, Kobara H, et al. Efficacy and safety of over-the-scope clip: including complications after endoscopic submucosal dissection. World J Gastroenterol 2013;19(18):2752–60. http://dx.doi.org/10.3748/wjg.v19.i18.2752.
27. Choi HS, Chun HJ, Kim ES, et al. Endoscopic suturing closure of large mucosal defects after endoscopic submucosal dissection: is the technique, at all times, feasible and effective? Gastrointest Endosc 2014;80(2):362–3. http://dx.doi.org/10.1016/j.gie.2014.03.003.
28. Fujihara S, Mori H, Kobara H, et al. Current innovations in endoscopic therapy for the management of colorectal cancer: from endoscopic submucosal dissection to endoscopic full-thickness resection. Biomed Res Int 2014;2014:925058. http://dx.doi.org/10.1155/2014/925058.
29. Kim HS, Kim TI, Kim WH, et al. Risk factors for immediate postpolypectomy bleeding of the colon: a multicenter study. Am J Gastroenterol 2006;101(6):1333.
30. Nelson DB, Freeman ML. Major hemorrhage from endoscopic sphincterotomy: risk factor analysis. J Clin Gastroenterol 1994;19(4):283.
31. Verma D, Kapadia A, Adler DG. Pure versus mixed electrosurgical current for endoscopic biliary sphincterotomy: a meta-analysis of adverse outcomes. Gastrointest Endosc 2007;66(2):283–90.

Foregut and Colonic Perforations

Practical Measures to Prevent and Assess Them

Jason N. Rogart, MD, FASGE

KEYWORDS

• Perforation • Colonoscopy • Endoscopy • Complication • Foregut • Colon

KEY POINTS

- Foregut and colonic perforations are rare adverse events during upper endoscopy or colonoscopy, but can cause significant morbidity and mortality when they occur.
- The endoscopist can take several measures to minimize the risk of procedure-related foregut and colonic perforations.
- A high index of suspicion is necessary for early, accurate, and thorough assessment of foregut and colonic perforations.
- Early diagnosis and assessment of perforations is critical in improving complication-related patient outcomes.

GENERAL PRINCIPLES: PREVENTION OF ACUTE ENDOSCOPIC PERFORATIONS

Like death and taxes, iatrogenic bowel perforation is a near certainty at some point during the life of a gastrointestinal (GI) endoscopist. Even the most skilled endoscopist who adheres to all of the principles of prevention will almost certainly face a situation whereby he or she has caused a foregut or colon perforation during endoscopy. Therefore, one should more realistically think of the clinical principles and pearls presented in this article as approaches to minimizing risk, as the only guaranteed way to avoid a perforation is to not perform the endoscopy at all.

Minimizing Risk of Perforation: General Principles

- Is the endoscopy indicated?
- Be prepared
- Know your limits
- Institute ongoing quality improvement programs

Capital Health Center for Digestive Health, Two Capital Way, Suite 380, Pennington, NJ 08534, USA

E-mail address: jrogart@capitalhealth.org

Gastrointest Endoscopy Clin N Am 25 (2015) 9–27
http://dx.doi.org/10.1016/j.giec.2014.09.004
1052-5157/15/$ – see front matter © 2015 Elsevier Inc. All rights reserved.

giendo.theclinics.com

Box 1
Frequency of acute endoscopic perforations

- Esophagogastroduodenoscopy: 0.05% to 0.1%

- Colonoscopy: 0.01% to 0.3%

- Endoscopic ultrasonography: 0% to 0.4%

- Endoscopic retrograde cholangiopancreatography: 0.5% to 1.5%

Perforation rates higher for more advanced therapeutic interventions.

Acute endoscopic perforations are, fortunately, a rare adverse event (**Box 1**).[1–7] When they do occur, however, they typically instill a great amount of fear in the endoscopist because of their potential to not only result in substantial morbidity and mortality, including sepsis and the need for surgery, but also strain the patient-physician relationship. The goal of this article is to assist in mitigating these fears by providing the endoscopist with practical measures to reduce the risk of iatrogenic foregut and colon perforations, and to discuss the appropriate means of assessing perforations when they inevitably occur.

Before every endoscopic procedure, the endoscopist should ask himself or herself, "Is this procedure truly indicated?" Though an obvious question, it should be answered from the perspective of not only the endoscopist but also the patient.

Next, it is important for the endoscopist to be prepared for the task at hand, whether that be resecting a polyp, dilating a stricture, or performing a sphincterotomy. Preparation includes several factors: (1) know the patient's history, in addition to any underlying comorbidities and medications that increase the risk for perforation (eg, connective tissue disorder, chronic steroid use); (2) schedule the procedure for the appropriate amount of time (eg, 30 minutes may not be reasonable for endoscopic mucosal resection of a large colon adenoma); (3) have expert mastery of the endoscopic equipment and devices that will be used, including their Food and Drug Administration–approved uses, how they work, and troubleshooting them when they malfunction. It is equally important that the staff (eg, nurses, technicians) in the room also have proficiency using the equipment and devices including, but is not limited to, operation of electrosurgical generators and their different settings, the characteristics of different snares, the differences in deploying different brands of endoclips, setting up band ligators, and use of devices or equipment that may be used infrequently such as polyvinyl endoloops or mechanical lithotripters. Some suggestions for ensuring that physicians and staff remain up to date and proficient in handling endoscopic equipment include working with representatives of the various device manufacturers to arrange for regular, periodic "in-services" where hands-on demonstrations and instructions are provided in detail; encouraging staff to attend conferences or hands-on workshops geared toward GI nurses and technicians; and creating specialized nurse/technician teams to regularly staff the more advanced cases that use unique equipment (eg, endoscopic retrograde cholangiopancreatography [ERCP], endoscopic ultrasonography [EUS], luminal stenting, GI bleeding).

Minimize Risk by Being Prepared

- Review patient's history and medications immediately before case
  - Identify any risk factors for perforation
- Schedule endoscopy for appropriate amount of time; do not rush

- Know the endoscopic equipment extremely well
  - Principles of electrosurgical generators
  - Devices
  - Troubleshooting when problems arise
- Ensure adequate training of nurses and technicians in equipment use
  - Hands-on "in-services" in endoscopy unit
  - Encourage attendance at educational conferences/workshops
  - Consider creating specialized nurse/technician teams to staff advanced cases (eg, interventional team for EUS/ERCP, GI bleeding team)

Even the best-prepared endoscopists, however, should know their capabilities and their limitations. Such knowledge will minimize the risk of perforation from maneuvers for which the endoscopist is inadequately trained or skilled in performing. For example, the decision may be made to refer a large, complicated colon polyp to a therapeutic endoscopist at a tertiary center. By doing so, the risk of perforation by both the referring physician and the endoscopist who will eventually perform the endoscopic mucosal resection can be reduced. Directors of endoscopy units can refer to published guidelines suggesting appropriate credentialing criteria.[8–10]

Knowing your Capabilities and Limitations will Reduce Risk

- Adequate training in procedure or maneuver being attempted
- Consider additional training at focused workshops, or a fourth-year advanced endoscopy fellowship
- Appropriate endoscopy unit credentialing/noncore privileging
- Know when to refer to a tertiary center

Finally, GI endoscopists and endoscopic units as a whole should participate in 1 or more programs focusing on ongoing practice performance (quality) improvement. For example, this may take the form of tracking adverse events and presenting them in hospital morbidity and mortality conferences, or comparing them with peers across the country via a database system such as the GI Quality Improvement Consortium (GiQuIC),[11] attending hospital morbidity and mortality conferences, and/or enrolling in the American Society for Gastrointestinal Endoscopy (ASGE) Endoscopic Unit Recognition Program.[12] By focusing on metrics of quality, including adverse events such as perforation, patterns and trends can be identified early so that a process to identify the etiology of a high perforation rate, for example, can be initiated, and a means to remediate the problem implemented.

Quality Improvement Programs can Reduce Risk

- Tracking perforation rates and comparing with peers (eg, GiQuIC)
- Attending hospital morbidity and mortality (M&M) conferences or practice performance committees
- GI society quality improvement courses
- ASGE Endoscopic Unit Recognition Program

GENERAL PRINCIPLES: ASSESSMENT OF ACUTE ENDOSCOPIC PERFORATIONS

Despite the best intentions and efforts, iatrogenic endoscopic perforations will occur. When they do occur, it is essential that the endoscopist knows how to assess and confirm the presence and location of a perforation, in addition to its severity. By doing so, the appropriate measures can be promptly taken, whether by attempting endoscopic closure, choosing to manage it conservatively with antibiotics, or calling a surgical colleague.

Early recognition of acute perforations is essential in improving the patient's outcome.[13] This recognition typically begins during the endoscopy by maintaining a high index of suspicion (**Fig. 1**). Perforation may be obvious, as when serosal fat is seen after resecting a large polyp in the colon. Other times, however, only subtle clues may be present such as difficulty in maintaining air insufflation, manifested by inability to keep the lumen of the bowel distended. Prompt recognition can allow for attempts at endoscopic closure and avoid potential sepsis, peritonitis, and the need for surgery.

Many times, however, a perforation is not appreciated at the time of endoscopy, and the patient may present with obvious symptoms such as abdominal pain and peritoneal abdominal signs on examination, or with vague, nonspecific symptoms or signs such as respiratory distress, confusion, or tachycardia (**Fig. 2**). In these situations, it is critical that the endoscopist has a low threshold for additional testing to evaluate for a possible perforation.

Imaging plays an important role in the postprocedure assessment of a perforation. Often the quickest and least expensive option is a plain radiograph of the chest and abdomen to evaluate for pneumothorax, pneumomediastinum, and free air under the diaphragm. Although retroperitoneal air can sometimes be seen, a computed tomography (CT) scan is a much more sensitive test if a retroperitoneal perforation is suspected (eg, after endoscopic biliary sphincterotomy). CT is also more sensitive for smaller perforations or microperforations and leaks; the approximate sensitivity and specificity of CT for perforation of the GI tract is 80% to 100%.[14,15] It is important to recognize, however, that extraluminal air on imaging is not always an indication for surgery.[16–18] The location, size, fluid collections, and clinical status of the patient all play a role in deciding whether a patient should be brought to the operating room,

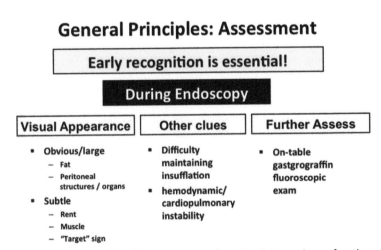

Fig. 1. General principles for the assessment of acute, iatrogenic perforations during endoscopy.

General Principles: Assessment

Post-Procedure

Symptoms	Signs

- Chest and/or abdominal pain
- Abdominal distension
- Respiratory distress
- Nausea/vomiting
- Confusion*
- Neck/scrotal swelling*

- Hypotension
- Tachycardia
- Hypoxia
- Subq crepitus
- Pneumothorax
- Fever
- Leukocytosis*

*typically manifests >24 hrs

Fig. 2. General principles for assessment of acute, iatrogenic perforation following completion of endoscopy.

although a surgical consultation should almost always be obtained in these situations. Two important principles to remember when extraluminal air is seen are: (1) air itself does not necessarily imply infection; and (2) the volume of free air is does not indicate the size of perforation, and is due in large part to the duration of the procedure and the volume of air insufflated after the perforation has occurred.[19,20] Location-specific approaches to assessing perforations are described in the following sections.

ESOPHAGEAL PERFORATIONS
Etiology

The overall reported rate of esophageal perforations during standard upper endoscopy is less than 0.1%. Perforation may rarely occur at the level of the hypopharynx or proximal esophagus from blind passage of the endoscope. This occurrence is more frequent with scopes that do not have a forward-viewing lens such as a duodenoscope (side-viewing) or echoendoscope (oblique-viewing).[21] Patients who are at higher risk for perforations in this location from scope passage, even with a forward-viewing endoscope, include those with Zenker diverticulum,[22] head and neck cancer, and prior external beam radiation therapy.

Therapeutic interventions carry a slightly higher risk of perforation even in experienced hands. Dilation of esophageal strictures with either a tapered-tip bougie or Savary dilator or a balloon catheter carries a risk of perforation of approximately 0.4%.[23,24] This rate may be higher in radiation-induced strictures,[25] and is higher in complicated (long and/or tortuous) strictures. Passage of a scope through a stricture, even without dilation, may also result in perforation, particularly if the scope is an echoendoscope or duodenoscope whereby the stricture may be unknown (if a standard esophagogastroduodenoscopy [EGD] was not performed first) or poorly visualized. In patients with foreign bodies or food impactions, there may be underlying strictures that can lead to perforations when endoscopy is performed. Pneumatic dilation of patients with achalasia carries a reported median risk of perforation of 2% to 4%.[24,26] Endoscopic mucosal resection (EMR) of mucosal lesions (nodules in Barrett esophagus) and subepithelial lesions are other causes of acute perforation. Esophageal stents can cause perforation at the time of stent insertion, or can occur much later if pressure necrosis occurs at the site of the stricture, or either end of a large stent; this can result in frank pneumomediastinum, or in the creation of respiratory esophageal fistulas.[27,28]

Causes of Endoscopic Esophageal Perforations

- Blind passage of endoscope (hypopharynx, proximal esophagus)
- Dilation of stricture
- Achalasia dilation
- Passage of non–forward-viewing endoscope through stricture
- Foreign body removal
- EMR of Barrett esophagus, intramucosal carcinoma, subepithelial lesions
- Long-standing esophageal stent

Assessment

If esophageal perforation is suspected at the time of endoscopy, visual inspection should be the first step in assessment. A perforation will appear as more than just a mucosal tear; often a defect in the muscle can be seen, or a frank hole may be obvious (**Fig. 3**). If there is uncertainty and the patient is in a room equipped with fluoroscopy, water-soluble contrast (eg, gastrograffin) can be injected through the scope during live fluoroscopy to determine whether there is any extraluminal extravasation of contrast. If a perforation is identified by any of the aforementioned methods, the endoscopist should assess whether it is small or large, its location, and whether it can be closed endoscopically (eg, with endoclips, over-the-scope clips, or endoscopic suturing), or sealed/occluded by placement of an esophageal stent.

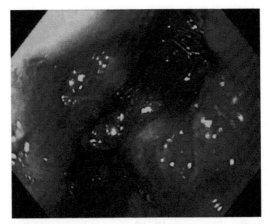

Fig. 3. Acute perforation of esophagus following balloon dilation of a benign stricture. The perforation can be visualized in the top right corner, whereas the esophageal lumen is seen at the bottom left corner. (*Courtesy of* Uzma Siddiqui, MD, University of Chicago, Chicago, IL.)

Many times the concern for esophageal perforation will occur in the immediate post-endoscopy period when the patient complains of chest or neck pain and may exhibit signs of respiratory distress or hemodynamic instability. Physical examination may reveal tachycardia, tachypnea, hypoxia, fever, and/or chest or neck crepitus. A plain radiograph of the chest may demonstrate air in the pleural space, mediastinum, or subcutaneous tissue. If this is seen, or further assessment is warranted, an esophagram with water-soluble contrast (not barium) or a CT scan of the chest with oral contrast should be obtained. Such imaging can identify the presence of a perforation as well as its location and approximate size.

Assessment of Iatrogenic Esophageal Perforations

Ways to assess:

- Visual inspection during endoscopy
- On-table fluoroscopic examination with water-soluble contrast
- Physical examination: tachycardia, tachypnea, hypotension, fever, chest or neck crepitus
- Plain chest radiograph
- Esophagram or chest CT

Goals of assessment:

- Identify presence, location, and size
- Determine if it can be closed or sealed endoscopically
- Determine if surgery is necessary

Prevention

Minimizing the risk of an esophageal perforation begins with careful passage of the endoscope past the hypopharynx and upper esophageal sphincter (UES), into the lumen of the esophagus. As mentioned earlier, this can be extremely challenging in certain subsets of patients (eg, Zenker diverticulum, cervical osteophytes, prior radiation therapy, complex strictures). Always maintaining the lumen in view and not pushing against resistance can help reduce the risk. With regard to passing ERCP or EUS endoscopes, this should be done only by those endoscopists who have had extensive training and are proficient in these procedures, as passing these scopes relies almost entirely on tactile feel. For the endosonographer, it is especially important to know when not to push too hard, as these scopes are larger and have less flexible tips. Performing a standard EGD immediately before EUS may help identify clinically significant lesions (ie, Zenker diverticulum, Shatzki ring, or unknown esophageal stricture), and thereby reduce the risk of perforation when inserting the echoendoscope.[29]

When dilating esophageal strictures, one should first assess the lumen diameter and then select the appropriate size and type of dilator needed. In the past, endoscopists anecdotally used the "rule of 3s" whereby no more than 3 successive sizes of dilators are used at one time once moderate resistance is encountered.[30] However, no studies have shown that this technique has improved safety outcomes.[31] If the stricture is long, tortuous, or complicated, one should also consider performing dilation under fluoroscopy and using wire-guided dilating catheters.[23] Alternatively, an ultraslim pediatric or transnasal endoscope may be used to traverse the stricture for a more complete assessment before dilation, and may negate the need for fluoroscopy. With regard to pneumatic dilation for achalasia, only endoscopists who have had formal training in this high-risk procedure should perform this operation. Lastly, patients should be counseled on the risks of delayed perforation or fistula formation with long-standing indwelling esophageal stents, particularly if they have a history of radiation therapy to the esophageal area, or a proximal stricture. For patients with proximal malignant strictures, it can be helpful to obtain a CT scan of the chest to assess for tracheal compromise or invasion, as this may increase the risk of stent-induced fistula formation.

Minimizing the Risk of Esophageal Perforations
- Careful passage of endoscope through hypopharynx and UES
- EUS and ERCP scopes should only be passed by those with experience
- Consider performing EGD before EUS
- Consider fluoroscopy for dilation of complicated strictures
- Proper patient selection for esophageal stent placement
- Beware leaving esophageal stents in place long term for benign disease

---

GASTRIC PERFORATIONS
Etiology

Compared with other locations within the GI tract, gastric perforations during endoscopy are extremely rare in the absence of underlying abnormality. The proximal stomach is at greatest risk, as this is where its wall is thinnest. The most common causes are related to the resection of mucosal or submucosal lesions during snare polypectomy, EMR, or endoscopic submucosal dissection (ESD). Perforation can also occur during dilation of surgical anastomotic strictures (eg, gastrojejunal anastomotic stricture in a patient who has undergone Roux-en-Y gastric bypass). Gastric perforation caused by a scope or barotrauma is fairly rare.

Causes of Endoscopy-Related Gastric Perforation
- Polypectomy
- EMR or ESD
- Dilation of anastomotic stricture
- Scope or barotrauma

Assessment

The principles of assessing for gastric perforations are similar to those described earlier for esophageal perforations. If possible, they should be identified during the endoscopy so that an attempt at endoscopic closure can be made (an easier feat in the stomach than in the esophagus). These perforations can appear, for example, as a defect in the muscle after EMR, yellow omental fat, or visualization of intraperitoneal organs or structures (**Fig. 4**). Inability to maintain a distended gastric lumen may be a clue that a perforation has occurred. If suspicion arises after the completion of the endoscopy or in the days ensuing, a thorough history, physical examination, laboratory testing, and appropriate imaging should be obtained, such as a CT scan of the abdomen and pelvis or upper GI series with water-soluble contrast (**Fig. 5**).

Assessment of Iatrogenic Gastric Perforations

Ways to assess:

- Visual inspection during endoscopy: defect in muscle; yellow fat
- Clue: inability to maintain distended gastric lumen with air insufflation
- Physical examination: hemodynamic or respiratory instability, fever, abdominal distension, peritoneal abdominal signs
- Imaging studies: Upper GI series with water-soluble contrast or CT scan of the abdomen and pelvis

Goals of assessment:

- Identify presence, location, and size
- Determine if it can be closed endoscopically
- Determine if surgery is necessary

Prevention

Though rare, perforation from scope trauma can be reduced by avoiding excessive looping in the stomach, which may occur during attempts to advance the gastroscope or enteroscope deep into the small bowel, or during attempts at advancing the duodenoscope to the major ampulla (especially in patients with surgically altered anatomy). Having the nurse or technician briefly apply left upper quadrant pressure can facilitate scope passage and minimize trauma from looping. Similarly, use of an overtube during enteroscopy can also decrease gastric loop formation. Many interventional endoscopists use carbon dioxide insufflation rather than air during invasive procedures such as those already mentioned, but it is unclear whether this reduces the risk of perforation or merely minimizes the clinical consequences if perforation occurs, as carbon dioxide is more rapidly absorbed than air.[32]

During resection of mucosal polyps or early gastric cancers, submucosal injection of saline or other substances to create a submucosal fluid cushion (SFC) that separates the mucosa/submucosa from the underlying muscularis propria can reduce the risk of perforation during use of snare cautery. Using endoclips or endoscopic sutures prophylactically after resection of large lesions or after ESD may also reduce the risk of perforation. When approaching subepithelial lesions (eg, carcinoid, pancreatic rest), initial evaluation with EUS is helpful in excluding those lesions that are not traditionally candidates for EMR (ie, those deeper than the submucosal layer). In addition, proper training in the use of cap-assisted EMR kits can reduce the risk of perforation. Just as for complicated esophageal strictures, the use of fluoroscopy during (at least the initial) dilation of an anastomotic surgical stricture can also minimize the risk of perforation.

Minimizing the Risk of Gastric Perforations

- Avoid excessive endoscope looping in the stomach; consider left upper quadrant pressure or use of overtube
- Submucosal injection of fluid before resecting large sessile lesions
- Perform EUS before resecting subepithelial lesions
- Proper training and use of cap-assisted EMR kit
- Consider use of fluoroscopy for dilating surgical gastric outlet strictures
- Consider use of carbon dioxide insufflation for therapeutic cases

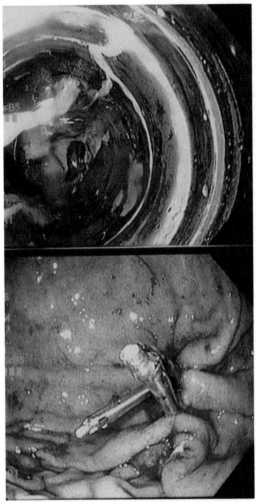

Fig. 4. After endoscopic mucosal resection (EMR) of a gastric subepithelial lesion was performed using a band-ligating EMR device, a 1-cm defect in the gastric wall is seen as well as an intraperitoneal structure (*top panel*). Because the perforation was recognized immediately, it was closed completely with endoclips (*bottom panel*).

DUODENAL PERFORATIONS
Etiology

Broadly speaking, duodenal perforations can be divided into nonampullary and ampullary related. The most common causes of nonampullary duodenal perforations include postpolypectomy or EMR. Carcinoid tumors may be at higher risk, although most of this evidence is anecdotal. Endotherapy for duodenal peptic ulcers can also result in perforation, particularly in deeply cratered ulcers when thermal therapy (eg, heater probe or bipolar cautery) is used. Dilation of duodenal strictures is also another cause of perforation; these are often more complicated than strictures encountered in the esophagus because they often occur in smaller spaces and difficult locations such as the duodenal sweep. Perforation of the duodenal sweep can also occur during passage of endoscopes, in particular echoendoscopes.

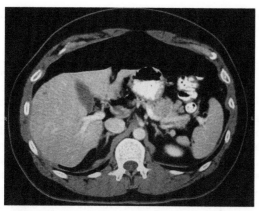

Fig. 5. Computed tomography scan of the abdomen performed for abdominal distension and discomfort following endoscopic mucosal resection of a gastric subepithelial lesion. A large amount of extraluminal free air in the ventral abdomen is seen.

Ampullary-related perforations typically occur during ERCP, and are discussed in detail in an article elsewhere in this issue. The duodenoscope, however, can cause duodenal perforations away from the ampulla. A typical location is at the contralateral duodenal wall from the elbow of the duodenoscope, which may not be recognized immediately. In addition, passage of the duodenoscope, with its side-viewing lens, may cause perforation in the small intestine of patients with altered anatomy (eg, Whipple or Billroth II).

Causes of Duodenal Perforation Occurring During Endoscopy

Nonampullary

- Polypectomy

- EMR

- Dilation of stricture

- Endotherapy for ulcers

- Passage of endoscope around duodenal sweep

- Trauma from ERCP duodenoscope (contralateral duodenal wall or post-Whipple/Bilroth II patients)

Ampullary (ERCP)

- Sphincterotomy

- Sphincteroplasty (large balloon dilation)

- Ampullectomy

Assessment

Along with other foregut perforations, assessment begins at the time of endoscopy with early recognition and assessment of whether endoscopic closure is feasible. During ERCP, for example, fluoroscopy can aid in identification by evaluating for retroperitoneal air or extravasation of contrast. After the procedure, upper GI series or CT scan of the abdomen and pelvis are the preferred imaging studies, as plain radiographs have a lower sensitivity for detection of retroperitoneal air.

Prevention

Prevention begins with careful advancement of the endoscope beyond the duodenal sweep. Likewise, when approaching patients with altered surgical anatomy, it is important to know what their current anatomy actually is (ie, what surgery they have undergone) before starting the endoscopy. During polypectomy or EMR, a robust SFC should be performed to separate the mucosal/submucosal layers from the muscularis propria. Avoiding capturing too much tissue in the snare can reduce the risk of perforation. En bloc movement of the duodenal wall along with the ensnared tissue can indicate a full-thickness ensnarement. When treating penetrating duodenal ulcers, cautiously delivering thermal therapy and using adjunctive methods of hemostasis (eg, epinephrine injection, hemoclips, over-the-scope clip) may reduce the risk of perforation.

During ERCP, using a proper technique during sphincterotomy (eg, cutting with the tip of the wire) and using caution (appropriately sized balloons to the duct diameter, slow inflation) during large balloon dilation can reduce the risk of ampullary-related perforations. This issue is discussed in more detail in an article elsewhere in this issue.

Reducing the Risk of Duodenal Perforations

- Careful passage of endoscope around duodenal sweep
- Know patient's anatomy if postsurgical
- Submucosal injection before resecting large mucosal lesions
- Supplemental nonthermal therapies for penetrating duodenal ulcers
- ERCP: proper sphincterotomy technique

COLORECTAL PERFORATIONS
Etiology

Most iatrogenic perforations during diagnostic colonoscopy occur in the rectum and sigmoid colon (53%) and cecum (24%), with the remainder evenly divided in the ascending, transverse, and descending colons.[33] The most common locations for perforations following therapeutic interventions, however, are the cecum and ascending colon, likely because of the thin wall and the technical challenges of resecting lesions in these locations.

During diagnostic colonoscopy, perforation can occur either from trauma induced by the tip of the colonoscope (eg, diverticula or navigating tight/angulated turns) or by the shaft of the colonoscope (eg, excessive looping or during retroflexion). Although it is logical to assume that polypectomy increases the risk of perforation, there are data from at least one study to suggest that standard polypectomy (<1 cm) does not have a higher risk than diagnostic colonoscopy.[34] Resection of larger polyps during EMR, however, clearly does increase the risk of perforation, and has been reported to be as high as 5% is some series.[35–37] Similarly, ESD of very large, laterally spreading sessile adenomas or early cancers has a reported risk of perforation of 5% to 10%.[36,38–40] Another cause of colorectal perforations is dilation of malignant strictures at the time of colonic stent insertion (7.4%).[41]

Causes of Endoscopic Colorectal Perforation

- Trauma from colonoscope
  - Tip diverticula, tight/angulated turns
  - Shaft looping, retroflexion
- Polypectomy (?)
- EMR
- ESD
- Coagulation of bleeding
- Dilation at the time of colonic stent placement

Assessment

Approximately one-third of colorectal perforations are recognized at the time of colonoscopy.[36] Visual inspection may reveal a mucosal rent, shiny-appearing serosa, epiploic fat, or free intraperitoneal space. The "target sign"[42] has also been recognized as a sign of probable perforation during polypectomy, particularly when blue dye is used in the SFC (eg, methylene blue or indigo carmine); this is manifested at the base of the resection site as a white center (muscularis propria) surrounded by pinkish or bluish tissue (dye-stained submucosa). Its mirror image can be seen on the underside of the resected specimen (**Figs. 6** and **7**). Recognition of this and other endoscopic clues at the time of colonoscopy is crucial to early management, as many of these can be treated endoscopically without the need for surgery.

If perforation is not recognized at the time of colonoscopy, symptoms of abdominal pain and/or distension (from pneumoperitoneum) typically occur within 24 hours. Fever, tachycardia, and hypotension can also ensue, as with any perforated viscus. A plain radiograph will typically show free air under the diaphragm, and a CT scan of the abdomen and pelvis may also show focal thickening of the colon at the site of perforation, in addition to pneumoperitoneum and potential fluid collections.

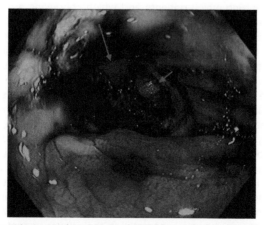

Fig. 6. After endoscopic mucosal resection of a large sigmoid sessile polyp, 2 sites of perforation are evident: epiploic fat seen through a hole (*long arrow*) and a "target sign" (*short arrow*). (*Courtesy of* Uzma Siddiqui, MD, University of Chicago, Chicago, IL.)

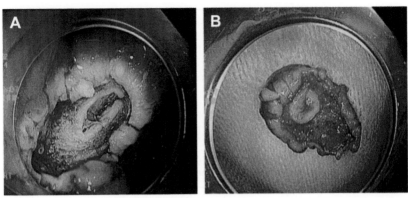

Fig. 7. Target sign after colon polypectomy (*A*) is suggestive of a perforation. The mirror image can be seen on the underside of the resected specimen (*B*).

In cases of rectal perforation, physical examination may show subcutaneous emphysema at distant sites such as the head, neck, and arms, owing to the continuum of facial planes. A CT scan may additionally show dissection of air through the perirectal tissues.

Signs of Colon or Rectal Perforation

- Endoscopic: mucosal rent, shiny serosa, fat, target sign
- Physical examination: abdominal distension and tenderness, distant subcutaneous emphysema (rectal)
- CT scan: pneumoperitoneum; thickening of colon at site of perforation; dissection of air through rectal tissues

---

Prevention

It may be possible to reduce the risk of perforation in patients undergoing colonoscopy by first recognizing which patients and which conditions are at higher risk, so that additional caution can be exercised (**Box 2**).[37,43–45]

Adequate visualization is probably the single most important factor in minimizing the risk of perforation. Pushing blindly through difficult areas will increase the likelihood of a perforation. In situations where there are tight turns (eg, adhesions, severe diverticulosis), a pediatric colonoscope or even a gastroscope should be considered if an adult colonoscope cannot be safely advanced. In addition, liberal use of water irrigation may provide lubrication or open the lumen enough to pass around difficult turns. If the bowel preparation is poor, one should consider aborting the case and rescheduling for another day. Poor bowel preparation not only decreases visualization but also can lead to fecal peritonitis if perforation occurs. Other ways to avoid scope trauma include minimizing excessive looping by using abdominal pressure from well-trained nurses or technicians, changing the position of the patient, or using specialized nonionizing imaging systems that can alert the endoscopist to looping on an external monitor (eg, Olympus ScopeGuide; Olympus America, Center Valley, PA, USA). Despite these measures, however, sometimes the cecum cannot be reached, and an alternative such as referral to an advanced endoscopist at a tertiary center or a CT colonography (virtual colonoscopy) should be considered.

Box 2
Risk factors for colonic perforation

- Severe diverticulosis
- Active severe colitis
- Elderly patients
- Adhesions from prior surgery
- Chronic steroid use
- Prior radiation therapy
- Large polyps
- Poor bowel preparation

Proper polypectomy technique will also reduce the risk of perforation in the colon and rectum. Hot biopsy forceps should no longer be used for resecting small polyps, owing to their relatively high perforation rate and the data showing that cold snare is safer.[46–48] When performing (hot) snare cautery, tenting the polyp away from the bowel wall will reduce the amount of transmural thermal injury. As in the duodenum, if there is en bloc movement of the colonic wall without obvious tenting, especially with a large amount of snared tissue, this can indicate a full-thickness ensnarement. For larger sessile polyps, an SFC is mandatory to limit thermal injury to the muscularis propria and ensure that the snare is not closed around the muscularis.[49] If all or a portion of the polyp cannot be raised with submucosal injection, one should be wary of proceeding with resection (nonlifting sign). In addition, there are data to suggest that performing piecemeal snare resection of polyps larger than 2 cm may reduce the risk of perforation compared with removing it en bloc in one piece, for reasons just mentioned.[50] Perhaps most importantly, one should know his or her own limitations with respect to colon polyp resection, and know when to refer a complex polyp to a therapeutic endoscopist who has had additional training and is proficient in EMR or ESD. The general gastroenterologist should only attempt polypectomy when he or she is certain that the polyp can be completely resected. Incomplete resection decreases the likelihood of the polyp being completely resected by a therapeutic endoscopist, and increases the risk of perforation during the subsequent attempt because of scarring.[51] The referring gastroenterologist should instead biopsy the edge of the polyp (if at all) and place an endoscopic tattoo away from the polyp. Biopsy of the center of the polyp or tattooing the lesion directly can cause submucosal fibrosis and may make it more difficult for the therapeutic endoscopist to completely resect it, and perhaps increase the perforation risk.

Lastly, with regard to the management of colon strictures, use of fluoroscopy and instillation of contrast can aid in a safer dilation. In addition, when placing colonic stents to treat colonic strictures, there are data suggesting that dilation done through the stent after deployment significantly increases the risk of perforation.[41]

Tips for Minimizing Risk of Colorectal Perforations

- Recognize patients/conditions at higher risk
- Visualize the lumen
  - Avoid pushing blindly
  - Use a smaller endoscope for severe diverticulosis or tight/sharp angulated colon

- o Use water irrigation liberally
- o Reschedule if bowel preparation is poor
- Avoid excessive colonoscope looping: abdominal pressure, position changes
- Avoid retroflexion in small rectum
- Consider carbon dioxide insufflation instead of air, especially in difficult cases
- Consider CT colonography rather than pushing past one's limits
- Use proper polypectomy technique
  - o Avoid hot biopsy forceps
  - o Tent polyp away from wall when using snare cautery
  - o Submucosal injection/lifting for larger sessile polyps
  - o Consider piecemeal resection if polyp larger than 2 cm
  - o Know when to refer to tertiary center for EMR (and do not attempt resection, biopsy the center of the polyp, or tattoo the polyp directly)
- Beware of dilating through colon stent after deployment

SUMMARY

Though rare, acute endoscopic perforations of the foregut and colon can have devastating consequences. Fortunately, the risk of perforation can be minimized by adequate endoscopic training, recognition of patients and conditions at increased risk for perforation, and knowing one's own limitations. When perforations do occur, however, patients' outcomes can be improved by early recognition and assessment so that endoscopic repair can be performed or appropriate medical and/or surgical management promptly initiated.

REFERENCES

1. Korman LY, Overholt BF, Box T, et al. Perforation during colonoscopy in endoscopic ambulatory surgical centers. Gastrointest Endosc 2003;58:554–7.
2. Wolfsen HC, Hemminger LL, Achem SR, et al. Complications of endoscopy of the upper gastrointestinal tract: a single-center experience. Mayo Clin Proc 2004; 79(10):1264–7.
3. Eloubeidi MA, Tamhane A, Varadarajulu S, et al. Frequency of major complications after EUS-guided FNA of solid pancreatic masses: a prospective evaluation. Gastrointest Endosc 2006;63:622–9.
4. Colton JB, Curran CC. Quality indicators, including complications, of ERCP in a community setting: a prospective study. Gastrointest Endosc 2009;70: 457–67.
5. Cotton PB, Garrow DA, Gallagher J, et al. Risk factors for complications after ERCP: a multivariate analysis of 11,497 procedures over 12 years. Gastrointest Endosc 2009;70:80–8.
6. Ko CW, Dominitz JA. Complications of colonoscopy: magnitude and management. Gastrointest Endosc Clin N Am 2010;20:659–71.
7. Hewitt MJ, McPhail MJ, Possamai L, et al. EUS-guided FNA for diagnosis of solid pancreatic neoplasms: a meta-analysis. Gastrointest Endosc 2012;75: 319–31.

8. ASGE Standards of Practice Committee, Eisen GM, Dominitz J, et al. Guidelines for credentialing and granting privileges for endoscopic ultrasound. Gastrointest Endosc 2001;54:811–4.

9. ASGE Standards of Practice Committee, Eisen GM, Dominitz J, et al. Principles of privileging and credentialing for endoscopy and colonoscopy. Gastrointest Endosc 2002;55:145–8.

10. ASGE Standards of Practice Committee, Dominitz JA, Ikenberry SO, et al. Renewal of and proctoring for endoscopic privileges. Gastrointest Endosc 2008;67:10–6.

11. Available at: http://giquic.gi.org. Accessed July 1, 2014.

12. Available at: http://www.asge.org/clinicalpractice/clinical-practice.aspx?id=13576. Accessed July 1, 2014.

13. La Torre M, Velluti F, Giuliani G, et al. Promptness of diagnosis is the main prognostic factor after colonoscopic perforation. Colorectal Dis 2012;14:e23–6.

14. Oguro S, Funabiki T, Hosoda K, et al. 64-Slice multidetector computed tomography evaluation of gastrointestinal tract perforation site: detectability of direct findings in upper and lower GI tract. Eur Radiol 2010;20:1396–403.

15. Cadenas Rodríguez L, Martí de Gracia M, Saturio Galán N, et al. Use of multidetector computed tomography for locating the site of gastrointestinal tract perforations. Cir Esp 2013;91:316–23.

16. Genzlinger JL, McPhee MS, Fisher JK, et al. Significance of retroperitoneal air after endoscopic retrograde cholangiopancreatography with sphincterotomy. Am J Gastroenterol 1999;94:1267–70.

17. Wiesen AJ, Sideridis K, Fernandes A, et al. True incidence and clinical significance of pneumoperitoneum after PEG placement: a prospective study. Gastrointest Endosc 2006;64:886–9.

18. Coriat R, Leblanc S, Pommaret E, et al. Transmural air leak following endoscopic submucosal dissection: a non-useful computed tomography finding. Endoscopy 2010;42:1117.

19. Enns R, Eloubeidi MA, Mergener K, et al. ERCP-related perforations: risk factors and management. Endoscopy 2002;34:293–8.

20. Fujii L, Lau A, Fleischer DE, et al. Successful nonsurgical treatment of pneumomediastinum, pneumothorax, pneumoperitoneum, pneumoretroperitoneum, and subcutaneous emphysema following ERCP. Gastroenterol Res Pract 2010;2010:289135.

21. ASGE Standards of Practice Committee, Early DS, Acosta RD, et al. Adverse events associated with EUS and EUS with FNA. Gastrointest Endosc 2013;77:839–43.

22. Case DJ, Baron TH. Flexible endoscopic management of Zenker diverticulum: the Mayo Clinic experience. Mayo Clin Proc 2010;85:719–22.

23. Hernandez LV, Jacobson JW, Harris MS. Comparison among the perforation rates of Maloney, balloon, and Savary dilation of esophageal strictures. Gastrointest Endosc 2000;51:460–2.

24. Katzka DA, Castell DO. Review article: an analysis of the efficacy, perforation rates and methods used in pneumatic dilation for achalasia. Aliment Pharmacol Ther 2011;34:832–9.

25. Swaroop VS, Desai DC, Mohandas KM, et al. Dilation of esophageal strictures induced by radiation therapy for cancer of the esophagus. Gastrointest Endosc 1994;40:311–5.

26. Vaezi MF, Pandolfino JE, Vela MF. ACG clinical guideline: diagnosis and management of achalasia. Am J Gastroenterol 2013;108:1238–49.

27. Sharma P, Kozarek R, Practice Parameters Committee of American College of Gastroenterology. Role of esophageal stents in benign and malignant diseases. Am J Gastroenterol 2010;105:258–73.
28. Varadarajulu S, Banerjee S, Barth B, et al, ASGE Technology Committee. Enteral stents. Gastrointest Endosc 2011;74:455–64.
29. Sahakian AB, Aslanian HR, Mehra M, et al. The utility of esophagogastroduodenoscopy before endoscopic ultrasonography in patients undergoing endoscopic ultrasonography for pancreatico-biliary and mediastinal indications. J Clin Gastroenterol 2013;47(10):857–60.
30. Langdon DF. The rule of three in esophageal dilation. Gastrointest Endosc 1997; 45:111.
31. Spechler SJ. AGA technical review on treatment of patients with dysphagia caused by benign disorders of the distal esophagus. Gastroenterology 1999; 117:233–54.
32. Maeda Y, Hirasawa D, Fujita N, et al. A pilot study to assess mediastinal emphysema after esophageal endoscopic submucosal dissection with carbon dioxide insufflation. Endoscopy 2012;44:565–71.
33. Iqbal CW, Cullinane DC, Schiller HJ, et al. Surgical management and outcomes of 165 colonoscopic perforations from a single institution. Arch Surg 2008;143: 701–6.
34. Warren JL, Klabunde CN, Mariotto AB, et al. Adverse events after outpatient colonoscopy in the Medicare population. Ann Intern Med 2009;150:849–57.
35. Repici A, Pellicano R, Strangio G, et al. Endoscopic mucosal resection for early colorectal neoplasia: pathologic basis, procedures, and outcomes. Dis Colon Rectum 2009;52:1502–15.
36. Raju GS, Saito Y, Matsuda T, et al. Endoscopic management of colonoscopic perforations (with videos). Gastrointest Endosc 2011;74:1380–8.
37. Buchner AM, Guarner-Argente C, Ginsberg GG. Outcomes of EMR of defiant colorectal lesions directed to an endoscopy referral center. Gastrointest Endosc 2012;76:255–63.
38. Tanaka S, Oka S, Kaneko I, et al. Endoscopic submucosal dissection for colorectal neoplasia: possibility of standardization. Gastrointest Endosc 2007; 66:100–7.
39. Niimi K, Fujishiro M, Kodashima S, et al. Long-term outcomes of endoscopic submucosal dissection for colorectal epithelial neoplasms. Endoscopy 2010;42: 723–9.
40. Saito Y, Uraoka T, Yamaguchi Y, et al. A prospective, multicenter study of 1111 colorectal endoscopic submucosal dissections (with video). Gastrointest Endosc 2010;72:1217–25.
41. van Halsema EE, van Hooft JE, Small AJ, et al. Perforation in colorectal stenting: a meta-analysis and a search for risk factors. Gastrointest Endosc 2014; 79:970–82.
42. Swan MP, Bourke MJ, Moss A, et al. The target sign: an endoscopic marker for the resection of the muscularis propria and potential perforation during colonic endoscopic mucosal resection. Gastrointest Endosc 2011;73:79–85.
43. Baxter NN, Tepper JE, Durham SB, et al. Increased risk of rectal cancer after prostate radiation: a population-based study. Gastroenterology 2005;128: 819–24.
44. Heldwein W, Dollhopf M, Rosch T, et al. The Munich Polypectomy Study (MUPS): prospective analysis of complications and risk factors in 4000 colonic snare polypectomies. Endoscopy 2005;37:1116–22.

45. Lohsiriwat V, Sujarittanakarn S, Akaraviputh T, et al. What are the risk factors of colonoscopic perforation? BMC Gastroenterol 2009;9:71.
46. Tappero G, Gaia E, De Giuli P, et al. Cold snare excision of small colorectal polyps. Gastrointest Endosc 1992;38:310–3.
47. Uno Y, Obara K, Zheng P, et al. Cold snare excision is a safe method for diminutive colorectal polyps. Tohoku J Exp Med 1997;183:243–9.
48. Metz AJ, Moss A, Mcleod D, et al. A blinded comparison of the safety and efficacy of hot biopsy forceps electrocauterization and conventional snare polypectomy for diminutive colonic polypectomy in a porcine model. Gastrointest Endosc 2013;77:484–90.
49. Soetikno R, Kaltenbach T. Dynamic submucosal injection technique. Gastrointest Endosc Clin N Am 2010;20:497–502.
50. Soetikno RM, Gotoda T, Nakanishi Y, et al. Endoscopic mucosal resection. Gastrointest Endosc 2003;57:567–79.
51. Moss A, Bourke MJ, Williams SJ, et al. Endoscopic mucosal resection outcomes and prediction of submucosal cancer from advanced colonic mucosal neoplasia. Gastroenterology 2011;140:1909–18.

Closing Perforations and Postperforation Management in Endoscopy
Esophagus and Stomach

Stavros N. Stavropoulos, MD*, Rani Modayil, MD, David Friedel, MD

KEYWORDS

- Perforation • Endoscopic closure • Through-the-scope clip • Over-the-scope clip
- Stent

KEY POINTS

- Endoscopic closure of perforations can be successfully achieved using a variety of devices.
- Even with endoscopic closure of perforations, the patient needs continued close monitoring with multidisciplinary input.
- Endoscopic closure of perforations effectively creates a leakproof seal, permits healing of perforation, prevents peritonitis, and limits peritoneal and mediastinal adhesions.

INTRODUCTION

Gastrointestinal luminal perforation may result from passage of the endoscope itself, diagnostic/therapeutic maneuvers (biopsy, dilation, ablation, polypectomy, endoscopic mucosal resection [EMR]/endoscopic submucosal dissection [ESD]), barotrauma (rare), or increasingly purposeful perforation, as in natural orifice transluminal endoscopic surgery (NOTES), including peroral endoscopic myotomy (POEM). Herein the authors emphasize endoscopic nonoperative management and their own and prior clinical experience in the literature, although animal studies are discussed regarding the rapidly evolving field of gastric perforation closure.

EPIDEMIOLOGY

A large retrospective analysis from the Mayo Clinic noted a perforation rate of 1 in 3000 upper endoscopy procedures, with a 38% higher rate with therapeutic

Disclosures: Dr S.N. Stavropoulos is a consultant for Boston Scientific. Drs R. Modayil and D. Friedel have no relevant disclosures.
Department of Gastroenterology, Hepatology and Nutrition, Winthrop University Hospital, 222 Station Plaza North, Suite 429, Mineola, NY 11501, USA
* Corresponding author.
E-mail address: sstavropoulos@winthrop.org

intervention.[1] Most of these perforations were esophageal (51%) and duodenal (32%), with only 3% gastric. The overall mortality was 17%, and 31% of deaths were related to esophageal perforations. Nearly half of these patients were treated nonoperatively; however, one-fifth of the patients failed nonoperative treatment within 3.7 days and required surgical intervention.[1] Meta-analysis of 75 studies of esophageal perforation yielded a pooled mortality of 17% and a mean hospital stay of 33 days.[2] The distal esophagus is the most common site in one review.[3] Gastric ESD is used for submucosal lesion resection and noninvasive neoplasia; one group noted a 5% perforation for the latter indication.[4]

GENERAL PRINCIPLES OF MANAGEMENT

There are several essential initial steps the endoscopist should consider after an actual or suspected upper gastrointestinal perforation. Most importantly, the endoscopist should remain calm because proper management may obviate surgical intervention. Prompt recognition of the perforation and patient positioning minimizes spillage outside the gastrointestinal tract and improves clinical outcomes.[5] Insufflation should be switched to carbon dioxide if room air is used initially. Endoscopic assessment is paramount, with attention to size, edge characteristics, and bleeding.[6] There are a variety of potential closure methods. Parenteral antibiotics and proton-pump inhibitors should be administered immediately and attention given to cardiopulmonary issues. Endotracheal intubation is advisable, although it should not delay closure attempt in an otherwise stable patient. Surgery (general/thoracic) should be notified and the patient triaged for intensive care unit monitoring.

Judicious use of radiologic examinations may be helpful after perforation, including after attempted closure. A lateral neck film may detect air after cervical esophageal perforation. Posterior and lateral chest and abdominal radiographs are ordered for more distal esophageal and gastric perforations. Contrast studies (eg, contrast esophagography to assess for esophageal perforation) using water-soluble agents (eg, gastrograffin) are valuable for diagnosing perforation, although occasionally perforations are missed because of technical considerations. Contrast may also be injected during endoscopy to assess perforation and degree of closure after intervention. Computed tomography (CT) is useful when traditional contrast studies are negative, and directs interventions such as drainage of collections. CT can demonstrate mediastinal and subcutaneous emphysema, pleural effusion, and pneumothorax. Patients with conservative treatment of perforations require vigilant clinical and radiographic follow-up.

The mere presence of extraluminal air does not mandate surgery, nor is the amount proportionate to perforation size.[7] On the other hand, air can dissect through tissue planes, and a compartment syndrome caused by air pressure is an emergency. Therefore, appropriate needles such as Veress needles or small-caliber angiocaths should be available to decompress tension pneumothorax and pneumoperitoneum. Needle insertion into the abdomen must be away from areas of potential organ injury (eg, away from surgical scars), and time must be allowed for adequate decompression. Failure to close an esophageal perforation usually mandates surgery. The stomach, on the other hand, is more "forgiving," and small gastric perforations may be amenable to conservative management. Gastric perforations usually benefit from nasogastric tube insertion for decompression and diversion of luminal contents. In some cases, nonoperative management may be considered in conjunction with interventional radiologic drainage.[7] Patients treated conservatively should keep fasting (nothing by mouth) with intravenous fluids and analgesia. Parenteral nutrition is considered, but selected patients should preferably receive enteral tube feedings distal to the pylorus if technically possible.

Endoscopic closure of esophageal, gastric, and colonic perforations, the subject of this review, has been investigated extensively in animal models. A recent review of these data concluded that the initial pilot studies and subsequent randomized controlled studies comparing endoscopic closure with surgical closure have demonstrated that "endoscopic closure of esophageal, gastric, and colon perforations is technically feasible, effective in creating a leak-proof closure, permits healing of perforation, prevents peritonitis, and limits peritoneal and mediastinal adhesions."[8] This review focuses mainly on clinical data from human studies pertaining to esophageal and gastric perforation closure.

ESOPHAGEAL PERFORATIONS
General Considerations

Esophageal perforation is encountered more commonly with therapeutic interventions such as stricture dilation, dilation for achalasia or eosinophilic esophagitis, foreign body extraction, or after ESD, but may also occur with diagnostic procedures such as a challenging esophageal intubation. Symptoms relate to site and extent of perforation and spillage of intraluminal contents. Subcutaneous emphysema is common. Neck pain is seen with cervical perforations, whereas severe chest pain, often with emesis, is noted with distal esophageal perforations. Fever, chills, tachycardia, and hypotension occur with development of sepsis.

Kuppusamy and colleagues[9] have demonstrated the evolution of esophageal perforation management over the past 20 years from surgery to nonoperative methods such as endoscopy and/or interventional radiology placed drains. Small esophageal perforations (<2 cm) can be closed with clips. Larger perforations usually require a covered self-expanding metal stent (SEMS). Perforations associated with distal obstruction arising from benign or malignant strictures or other conditions such as achalasia are also best served with a stent to alleviate high luminal pressures in the area of the perforation that may result in failure of endoscopic closure. Perforations with everted edges are especially challenging, and may be best treated with endoluminal suturing or large over-the-scope clips (OTSCs), although use of these devices can be challenging in the esophagus, especially the proximal esophagus, owing to space constraints.[10] Cervical esophageal perforations can often be treated conservatively because of containment by the neck fascial structures. This circumstance is fortunate because endoscopic closure of any type is difficult in the narrow tapered cervical esophagus, and patients are less tolerant of proximally deployed stents near the upper esophageal sphincter.

Clips

Through-the-scope (TTS) endoscopic mucosal clips can be used to close small perforations provided that the tissue surrounding the edges is compliant and viable. TTS clips are made by several companies and differ in terms of their diameter, rotation capacity, and deployment capability after multiple openings (**Fig. 1**). **Table 1** compares the key features of the more commonly used TTS clips. Occasionally they can be used to close larger, nongaping perforations. The endoscopist and assistant should be well versed with their chosen device, and coordinate their actions. Raju[10] recommends approaching a linear tear from above, with the first clip tenting up tissue near the top edge of the perforation, and approaching a circular perforation from below with intended transverse closure. In either instance, multiple clips are applied

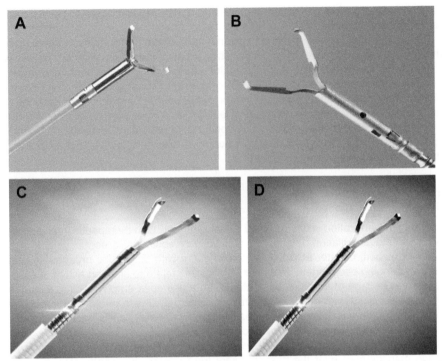

Fig. 1. (*A*) Instinct clip. (*B*) Resolution clip. (*C*) QuickClip. (*D*) QuickClip Pro. (*Courtesy of* [*A*] Cook Medical, Bloomington, IN, with permission; and [*B*] Boston Scientific, Natick, MA, with permission; [*C, D*] Olympus, Center Valley, PA, with permission.)

Table 1
Comparison of through-the-scope (TTS) endoscopic clipping devices

Characteristics	QuickClip2 QuickClip Pro (Olympus)	Resolution Clip (Boston Scientific)	Instinct Clip (Cook Medical)
Sheath diameter (F)	7 7	7	7
Sheath length (cm)	235 230	230	230
Jaw opening width (mm)	9, 11 11	11	16
Reopening and repositioning ability	No Yes	Yes	Yes
Rotating ability	Yes Yes	No	Yes
Clip material	Stainless steel Elgiloy	Stainless steel	Stainless steel and nitinol
Deployment	Two-step Three-step	Three step	Two step
MRI compatible	No Up to 3 T	Up to 3 T	Up to 3 T
Approximate cost ($, per clip)	65 Not available	170	150

in a parallel fashion to achieve closure. Enhancing maneuvers include orienting the clip in the intended position and simultaneously applying suction to invert and approximate the perforation edges, and only deploying the clip when the edges are approximated.[11] A double-channel endoscope can be also used, which allows for a long grasping forceps to be passed through one channel to grasp the edges and initiate the closure. Then a mucosal or TTS clip is used through the other channel parallel to the grasped tissue, alongside the grasper, with subsequent deployment of the clip.

There is limited literature supporting the use of TTS clips in the closure of esophageal perforations, and several series include noniatrogenic perforations in addition to leaks and fistulas.[11] **Table 2** summarizes published case reports and case series describing successful esophageal perforation closure with endoscopic mucosal clips. TTS closure has been shown to be successful in a variety of circumstances including EMR, Boerhaave syndrome, and balloon-, tube-, and endoscope-related perforation, without the need for prolonged hospitalization.

An OTSC (Ovesco, Tübingen, Germany) was developed for closure of mural defects up to 18 mm in size and bleeding ulcers (**Fig. 2**).[20] The device comes in various sizes, includes a large-caliber nitinol clip that fits over a cap at the tip of the endoscope, and is deployed in similar fashion to bands from a variceal ligator. The OTSC has been successfully deployed throughout the gastrointestinal tract. **Table 3** summarizes published case reports and case series describing successful esophageal perforation closure with OTSCs. In a European multicenter prospective cohort study, all 5 patients with esophageal perforations had successful closure with the OTSC.[21] Ironically, in this study 1 patient with a duodenal perforation sustained an esophageal perforation with insertion of the device. In other series, 3 patients with esophageal perforation had successful OTSC closure.[22] There has also been mention of successful closure of esophageal perforation caused by nasogastric tube placement with OTSC.[23] Hagel and colleagues[24] reviewed the predictors of successful use of the OTSC, and found

Table 2		
Published literature on endoscopic clip closure of esophageal perforation		
TTS Clip Closure of Esophageal Perforations	**Type of Study**	**Comments**
Shimizu et al,[12] 2004	Case series	3 patients after EMR: successfully closed
Qadeer et al,[3] 2007	Case report and pooled analysis	Pooled analysis: 11 articles with 17 patients: median healing time = 18 d Success diminished with chronicity
Gerke et al,[13] 2007	Case report	Proximal perforation caused by diagnostic EGD. Successful closure
Fischer et al,[14] 2007	Case series	2 diagnostic, 1 dilation, 1 laser. All successfully closed
Mangiavillano et al,[15] 2010	Pooled analysis	10 patients: all successfully closed
Rokszin et al,[16] 2011	Case report	Boerhaave syndrome: no surgery required
Jung et al,[17] 2011	Case report	Blakemore tube insertion complication: no surgery required
Coda et al,[18] 2012	Case report	After achalasia balloon dilation: no surgery required
Huang et al,[19] 2014	Case series	Esophageal perforation caused by duodenoscope: all successfully closed

Abbreviations: EGD, esophagogastroduodenoscopy; EMR, endoscopic mucosal resection.

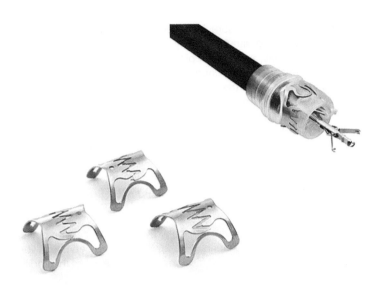

Fig. 2. Over-the-scope clip (OTSC or "bear claw"). (*Courtesy of* Ovesco, Los Gatos, CA, with permission.)

that perforations located in the proximal and mid esophagus, greater than 20 mm in size, with ischemic or inflamed margins or present for greater than 72 hours, were least amenable to OTSC closure.

Stents

As already mentioned, endoscopic esophageal stenting is an effective means of closing larger esophageal perforations because it minimizes unfavorable pressure gradients related to strictures and achalasia that may cause an endoscopic closure to fail. Care should be taken to center the stent after deployment on the perforation

Table 3
Published literature on over-the-scope clip (OTSC) closure of esophageal perforations

OTSC Closure of Esophageal Perforations	N	Technical/ Clinical Success (%)	Other Treatments	Complications
Kirschniak et al,[25] 2011	7	100/100	—	—
Baron et al,[26] 2012	1	100/100	—	—
Voermans et al,[21] 2012	5	100/100	Adjunctive clips and second OTSC	—
Hagel et al,[24] 2012	4	25 (1/4)	Surgical suture	Enlargement of perforation
Haito-Chavez et al,[27] 2014	10	100/100	—	—
Jacobsen et al,[22] 2012	3	100/100	—	—
Nishiyama et al,[23] 2013	1	100/100		
Ramhamadany et al,[28] 2013	1	100/100	—	—
Ferreira et al,[29] 2013	1	100/100	—	—
Bona et al,[30] 2014	1	100/100	—	—

site. Stents are less optimal in the proximal esophagus (foreign body sensation) and with a previously normal gastroesophageal junction (gastroesophageal reflux disease and migration). There had been some initial work with a plastic expandable stent (Polyflex; Boston Scientific, Natick, MA, USA), which was found to have unacceptably high migration rates. Most recent published experience has been predominantly with covered SEMS. These stents are made by several different companies and come in a variety of dimensions, radial forces, and mechanisms of deployment and removal. There is also a biodegradable stent, although it is not currently available in the United States (Ella-CS, Hradec Králové, Czech Republic).[31]

Table 4 summarizes published series describing successful esophageal perforation closure with stents. Some have advocated smaller-diameter stents for more proximal perforations.[11] There are insufficient data to suggest superiority of any particular expandable metal stent. Optimally, they are inserted with both endoscopic and fluoroscopic guidance.[11] Migration represents a significant problem and is one of the main causes of failure. Attempts to secure these stents against migration have included fixation of the stents with clips, endoscopic sutures, or even a bridle,[32–34] the latter 2 methods probably representing more reliable fixation than can be achieved with TTS clips.

Four patients with esophageal perforation had technically successful closure with a removable plastic stent, but 1 patient died secondary to malignancy and stent migration was seen in 30% of patients.[36] Migration appears to occur at a higher rate with fully covered metal stents and the least with partially covered metal stents, although the latter may be more challenging to remove.[11] In a series of 22 patients (9 with esophageal cancer) with esophageal perforation or leak who received a partially covered metal stent (Ultraflex; Boston Scientific), all but 1 had technical success (closure), but 5 patients died (3 from perforation complications).[37] Fifteen patients without malignancy had esophageal perforations treated with partially covered SEMS with 100% technical success (closure), but 1 person died of pneumonia at 6 days postoperatively, and the group of patients with somewhat delayed stent insertion had increased morbidity and prolonged hospital stay.[38] A recent systematic review of 27 case series including an aggregate number of 340 patients noted technical and clinical success of 91% and 81%, respectively.[48] Despite this ample supportive literature on esophageal stenting for esophageal perforation there remains skepticism, especially among surgeons, with one recent review concluding that the utility of stenting is "unproven and controversial."[49]

Other Therapies

Endoscopic vacuum-assisted closure (EVAC) uses negative pressure to absorb secretions and promote wound healing by secondary intention.[50] EVAC has demonstrated significant efficacy (>90%) in several case series.[11,50] The endoscopic suturing system (OverStitch; Apollo Endosurgery, Austin, TX, USA) is a disposable single-use suturing device (**Fig. 3**)[33] that allows either running or interrupted full-thickness sutures. Esophageal perforation has been sutured closed, but experiences are limited. OverStitch has been used to secure stents and close perforations during POEM.[33,51] Use of fibrin glue has also been reported for closure of esophageal perforations secondary to POEM.[52]

GASTRIC PERFORATIONS
General Considerations

Gastric perforation is extremely rare without instrumentation and, until recently, an uncommon endoscopic complication.[1] Occasionally it is encountered with transgastric

Table 4
Published literature on stent closure of esophageal perforations

Study	No. of Perforations	Stent	Migration (%)	Mortality (%)	Clinical Success (%)
Siersema et al,[35] 2003	8	Flamingo/Ultraflex	9	0	93
Gelbmann et al,[36] 2004	4	Polyflex	30	33	66
Johnsson et al,[37] 2005	20	Ultraflex	14	23	77
Fischer et al,[38] 2006	15	Ultraflex/Niti S	—	7	93
Ott et al,[39] 2007	4	Polyflex	33	50	50
Freeman et al,[40] 2007	17	Polyflex/Wallflex	18	0	94
Tuebergen et al,[41] 2008	10	Ultraflex	6	15	81
Kim et al,[42] 2008	9	Salivary bypass	35	11	77
Leers et al,[43] 2008	9	Ultraflex	3	0	100
Kiev et al,[44] 2007	9	Polyflex	21	0	100
Salminen et al,[45] 2009	8	Ultraflex	10	30	70
van Heel et al,[46] 2010	31	Ultraflex/Polyflex	33	15	74
Kuppusamy et al,[6] 2011	52	Polyflex/Wallflex/Niti S	21	0	100
Dai et al,[47] 2011	6	Polyflex	35	17	83

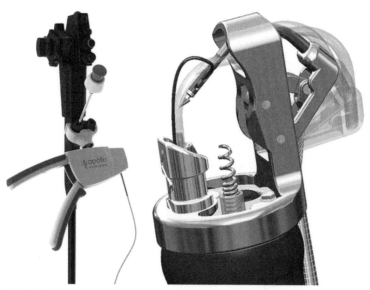

Fig. 3. OverStitch endoscopic suturing system. (*Courtesy of* Apollo Endosurgery, Austin, TX)

drainage of fluid collections and dilation of gastroenteric anastomoses. The advent of ESD (and to a lesser extent EMR) and NOTES has changed this paradigm, as gastric perforation is a complication encountered not infrequently by those performing ESD for early gastric neoplasia or subepithelial tumors, and gastric perforation is in fact an intentional step of NOTES interventions such as endoscopic full-thickness resection (EFTR) for complete R0 resection of deep-seated subepithelial tumors such as gastrointestinal stromal tumors.

Carbon dioxide must be used during endoscopy before gastric EMR/ESD in anticipation of possible perforation. Appropriate needles, such as a Veress needle for decompression of pneumoperitoneum, should also be available. Antibiotics, generous fluids, and proton-pump inhibitors should be administered intravenously in the event of gastric perforation. The stomach should be well suctioned via the endoscope before embarking on a resection, and optimally the patient should be positioned so that gravity drains gastric contents away from a site of possible perforation. Many of the already mentioned technical considerations for clip closure can also apply to the stomach; especially the need for well-approximated perforation edges. The stomach, fortunately, is the most resilient and robust organ after perforation, as evidenced from likely closure of a gastrocutaneous fistula after percutaneous endoscopic gastrostomy.[7]

Clips

TTS clips are the mainstay of closure of gastric perforations, and have an excellent track record. **Table 5** summarizes published series describing successful gastric perforation closure with mucosal clips. Minami and colleagues[53] published the largest series of postresection gastric perforations. A total of 121 out of 2460 patients (4.9%) who underwent gastric EMR or ESD sustained perforation, of whom 115 (98.3%) had successful mucosal clip closure with only 4 patients needing emergency surgery. There was a predilection for a higher proportion of perforations in the proximal stomach; perhaps because of differences of wall thickness in comparison with the antrum (**Fig. 4**). A recent gastric ESD series (for noninvasive gastric neoplasia) had a similar

Table 5
Published literature on endoscopic clip closure of gastric perforations

Study (Year)	N	Etiology	Technical/Clinical Success (%)	Other Treatment for Failures	Mortality	Comments
Tsunada et al,[55] 2003	7	EMR	100/100	—	0	
Minami et al,[53] 2006	117	EMR, ESD	98.3/98.3	Surgery	0	Closure failed because of severe bleeding and clinical deterioration. Omental patch used for defect >1 cm
Fujishiro et al,[56] 2006	11	ESD	100/100	—	0	
Imagawa et al,[57] 2006	12	ESD	100/100	—	0	
Jeon et al,[58] 2010	26	ESD	96.1/96.1	Surgery	0	Closure failed because of severe bleeding and clinical deterioration
Toyokawa et al,[54] 2012	27	ESD	96.3/96.3	Surgery	0	Large tumor in cardia and clinical deterioration (severe dyspnea from pneumothorax and pneumomediastinum)
Zhang et al,[60] 2013	32	ESD	100/100	—	0	Higher perforation rate in body and fundus than antrum
Li et al,[61] 2013	3	ESD	100/100	—	0	Successful closure of fundic perforations
He et al,[62] 2013	6	ESD	100/100	—	0	Used nylon band as adjunctive therapy

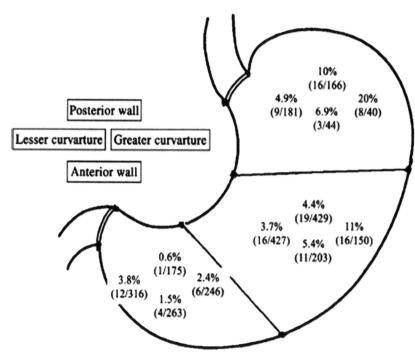

Fig. 4. Rates of gastric perforation according to aspect of gastric wall. (*From* Minami S, Gotoda T, Ono H, et al. Complete endoscopic closure of gastric perforation induced by endoscopic resection of early gastric cancer using endoclips can prevent surgery (with video). Gastrointest Endosc 2006;63(4):599; with permission.)

perforation rate (5.1%), with perforation being more likely with lesions of greater curvature.[4] Toyokawa and colleagues[54] examined ESD for more than 1000 gastric lesions (early gastric neoplasia) and encountered 27 perforations (2.4%) of which 26 were closed successfully, and noted that ESD in the proximal stomach was the only significant risk factor for perforation. The sole patient who needed surgery had a large cardiac lesion and developed pneumothorax and pneumomediastinum. However, overall there was no reported mortality from these and other gastric ESD series, and a very high rate of gastric perforation closure.

It should be noted, however, that accidental perforations arising from endoscopic resection are usually small (2–3 mm) defects caused by accidental transmural injury of the muscularis by the small monopolar instruments used during the resection. Therefore, closure by TTS clips for these resection-related perforations is easier than closure of large defects secondary to barotrauma or endoscope-tip puncture (rare occurrences) or EFTR of subepithelial neoplasms, an emerging NOTES technique. For such large defects simple clip closure has been described,[63] but this may be hard to achieve or may result in less secure closure than when TTS clips are used to close smaller perforations. Zhang and colleagues[59] described successful closure of EFTR defects in 30 patients by placing clips in the margins of the resection and then approximating the clips using an endoloop, effectively achieving a purse-string closure. Such endoloop plus TTS clips purse-string closure techniques, including so-called King's closure, Queen's closure, and double-endoloop technique, have been previously described for closure of gastric perforations, and compared in an animal model with OTSC closure of such perforations.[64–67]

Minami and colleagues[53] described an omental patch closure technique for closure of defects greater than 1 cm, whereby omentum and fat were purposefully drawn into the perforation defect before clip application to promote physiologic closure. This concept of omental patch closure is drawn from surgical treatment of gastroduodenal ulcer and a porcine model of gastric perforation.[68]

The OTSC has been demonstrated to close larger gastric perforations in both animal models and patients.[69,70] The clip comes in multiple sizes, and supplemental tools include 2 tissue-grasping devices (tissue anchor, twin grasper), which help approximate tissue and bring the edges of the defect within the cap at the tip of the endoscope to properly deploy the clip, so as to seal the defect. **Table 6** summarizes case reports and case series describing successful gastric perforation closure with OTSC. However, the device may be difficult to use in the proximal stomach.

Other Therapies

Endoscopic stents are not usually useful for gastric perforations, but may be useful to treat leaks following sleeve gastrectomy, pyloric or gastroenteric anastomosis dilation perforations, or with persistent perigastric air after transgastric pancreatic fluid plastic stent placement.[7] The endoscopic suturing device has successfully closed post-ESD defects.[73] Other suturing devices are in development, including one that has an external component of hand sutures applied outside the gastric wall.[74] One series described endoscopic band ligation for gastric perforation closure.[75]

NATURAL ORIFICE TRANSLUMINAL ENDOSCOPIC SURGERY

The Holy Grail of NOTES is reproducible, reliable, and durable closure of the gastric perforation after endoscopic entry into the peritoneal cavity. One concept uses a method referred to as submucosal endoscopy with a protective mucosal flap (SEMF). This method converts the submucosa into a working space or tunnel, allowing off-set entry into the peritoneal cavity at the distal end of the submucosal tunnel. The overlying mucosa serves as a sealant. The mucosal entry point can be easily closed with a variety of closures.[76] This technique has been used in POEM. There is intense animal laboratory work on NOTES gastric closure techniques, including endoscopic suturing, OTSCs, T-tags, and biological plugs.[77–80] It is likely that there will be several acceptable methods for closure of large gastric perforations in the future.

Table 6
Published literature on OTSC closure of gastric perforations

Study (Year)	N	Technical/Clinical Success	Other Treatments	Mortality
Schlag et al,[71] 2013	6	100/100	—	0
Baron et al,[26] 2012	2	100/100	—	0
Voermans et al,[21] 2012	6	100/100	Adjunctive clips and second OTSC	0
Hagel et al,[24] 2012	7	71 (5/7)	Surgical suture Endoloop closure, antibiotics, TPN, NG tube	0
Gubler et al,[72] 2012	3	66	Surgery	0
Nishiyama et al,[23] 2013	4	75/75	Surgery	0
Haito-Chavez et al,[27] 2014	13	100/100	—	0

Abbreviations: NG, nasogastric; TPN, total parenteral nutrition.

SUMMARY

Esophageal perforation is an inadvertent, potentially catastrophic endoscopic complication that will have dire consequences if not treated urgently. Historically it was considered a surgical issue, but the endoscopist now has a variety of options including stents, clips, and direct suturing that may negate the need for surgery. However, even with endoscopic closure, the patient remains critically ill, and continued close monitoring is required with multidisciplinary input. Gastric perforation is increasingly encountered with the increasing use of gastric ESD and other resection techniques. Closure methods are readily available, usually achieving excellent results. There is significant animal research focusing on novel techniques for closure of large perforations, particularly those associated with NOTES procedures, such as EFTR.

REFERENCES

1. Merchea A, Cullinane DC, Sawyer MD, et al. Esophagogastroduodenoscopy-associated gastrointestinal perforations: a single-center experience. Surgery 2010;148(4):876–80.
2. Biancari F, Saarnio J, Mennander A, et al. Outcome of patients with esophageal perforations: a multicenter study. World J Surg 2014;38(4):902–9.
3. Qadeer MA, Dumot JA, Vargo JJ, et al. Endoscopic clips for closing esophageal perforations: case report and pooled analysis. Gastrointest Endosc 2007;66(3): 605–11.
4. Ojima T, Takifuji K, Nakamura M, et al. Complications of endoscopic submucosal dissection for gastric noninvasive neoplasia: an analysis of 647 lesions. Surg Laparosc Endosc Percutan Tech 2014;24:370–4.
5. Vallböhmer D, Hölscher AH, Hölscher M, et al. Options in the management of esophageal perforation: analysis over a 12-year period. Dis Esophagus 2010; 23(3):185–90.
6. Kuppusamy MK, Felisky C, Kozarek RA, et al. Impact of endoscopic assessment and treatment on operative and non-operative management of acute oesophageal perforation. Br J Surg 2011;98(6):818–24.
7. Baron TH, Wong Kee Song LM, Zielinski MD, et al. A comprehensive approach to the management of acute endoscopic perforations. Gastrointest Endosc 2012; 76(4):838–59.
8. Raju GS. Gastrointestinal perforations: role of endoscopic closure. Curr Opin Gastroenterol 2011;27(5):418–22.
9. Kuppusamy MK, Hubka M, Felisky CD, et al. Evolving management strategies in esophageal perforation: surgeons using nonoperative techniques to improve outcomes. J Am Coll Surg 2011;213(1):164–71 [discussion: 171–2].
10. Raju G. Endoscopic closure of leaks, fistulas and perforations. Retrieved from ASGE News. Available at: http://www.asge.org/uploadedFiles/ASGE_News/ AENov09.pdf. 1–4. Accessed June 1, 2014.
11. Yuan J, Baichoo E, Song L. Endoscopic therapies for acute perforations and leaks. Tech Gastrointest Endosc 2001;16(1):53–61.
12. Shimizu Y, Kato M, Yamamoto J, et al. Endoscopic clip application for closure of esophageal perforations caused by EMR. Gastrointest Endosc 2004;60(4): 636–9.
13. Gerke H, Crowe GC, Iannettoni MD. Endoscopic closure of cervical esophageal perforation caused by traumatic insertion of a mucosectomy cap. Ann Thorac Surg 2007;84(1):296–8.

14. Fischer A, Schraq HJ, Goos M, et al. Nonoperative treatment of four esophageal perforations with hemostatic clips. Dis Esophagus 2007;20(5):444–8.
15. Mangiavillano B, Viaggi P, Masci E. Endoscopic closure of acute iatrogenic perforations during diagnostic and therapeutic endoscopy in the gastrointestinal tract using metallic clips: a literature review. J Dig Dis 2010;11(1):12–8.
16. Rokszin R, Simonka Z, Paszt A, et al. Successful endoscopic clipping in the early treatment of spontaneous esophageal perforation. Surg Laparosc Endosc Percutan Tech 2011;21(6):e311–2.
17. Jung JH, Kim JI, Song JH, et al. A case of Sengstaken-Blakemore tube-induced esophageal rupture repaired by endoscopic clipping. Intern Med 2011;50(18): 1941–5.
18. Coda S, Antonellis F, Tsagkaropulos S, et al. Complete endoscopic closure (clipping) of a large esophageal perforation after pneumatic dilation in a patient with achalasia. J Laparoendosc Adv Surg Tech A 2012;22(8):815–8.
19. Huang J, Wen W, Tang X, et al. Cap-assisted clip closure of large esophageal perforations caused by a duodenoscope during endoscopic retrograde cholangiopancreatography (with video). Surg Laparosc Endosc Percutan Tech 2014; 24(3):e101–5.
20. ASGE Technology Committee, Banerjee S, Barth BA, et al. Endoscopic closure devices. Gastrointest Endosc 2012;76(2):244–51.
21. Voermans RP, Le Moine O, Von Rentein D, et al. Efficacy of endoscopic closure of acute perforations of the gastrointestinal tract. Clin Gastroenterol Hepatol 2012; 10(6):603–8.
22. Jacobsen GR, Coker AM, Acosta G, et al. Initial experience with an innovative endoscopic clipping system. Surg Technol Inc 2012;22:39–53.
23. Nishiyama N, Mori H, Kobara H, et al. Efficacy and safety of over-the-scope clip: including complications after endoscopic submucosal dissection. World J Gastroenterol 2013;19(18):2752–60.
24. Hagel AF, Naegel A, Lindner AS, et al. Over-the-scope clip application yields a high rate of closure in gastrointestinal perforations and may reduce emergency surgery. J Gastrointest Surg 2012;16(11):2132–8.
25. Kirschniak A, Subotova N, Zieker D, et al. The over-the-scope clip (OTSC) for the treatment of gastrointestinal bleeding, perforations, and fistulas. Surg Endosc 2011;25(9):2901–5.
26. Baron TH, Song LM, Ross A, et al. Use of an over-the-scope clipping device: multicenter retrospective results of the first U.S. experience (with videos). Gastrointest Endosc 2012;76(1):202–8. http://dx.doi.org/10.1016/j.gie.2012.03.250.
27. Haito-Chavez Y, Law JK, Kratt T, et al. International multicenter experience with an over-the-scope clipping device for endoscopic management of GI defects (with video). Gastrointest Endosc 2014. http://dx.doi.org/10.1016/j.gie.2014.03. 049. pii:S0016–5107(14)01334-0.
28. Ramhamadany E, Mohamed S, Jaunoo S, et al. A delayed presentation of Boerhaave's syndrome with mediastinitis managed using the over-the-scope clip. J Surg Case Rep 2013;2013(5). pii:rjt020.
29. Ferreira AO, Lopes J, Velosa J. Snapper fishbone esophageal perforation closed with an over-the-scope-clip. BMJ Case Rep 2013;2013. pii:bcr2013201614.
30. Bona D, Aiolfi A, Rausa E, et al. Management of Boerhaave's syndrome with an over-the-scope clip. Eur J Cardiothorac Surg 2014;45(4):752–4.
31. Griffiths EA, Gregory CJ, Pursnani KG, et al. The use of biodegradable (SX-ELLA) oesophageal stents to treat dysphagia due to benign and malignant oesophageal disease. Surg Endosc 2012;26(8):2367–75.

32. Vanbiervliet G, Filippi J, Karimdjee BS, et al. The role of clips in preventing migration of fully covered metallic esophageal stents: a pilot comparative study. Surg Endosc 2012;26(1):53–9.

33. Fujii LL, Bonin EA, Baron TH, et al. Utility of an endoscopic suturing system for prevention of covered luminal stent migration in the upper GI tract. Gastrointest Endosc 2013;78(5):787–93.

34. Lyons CD, Kim MP, Blackmon SH. A novel fixation procedure to eliminate covered self-expanding metal stent migration. Ann Thorac Surg 2012;94(5):1748–50.

35. Siersema PD, Homs MY, Haringsma J, et al. Use of large-diameter metallic stents to seal traumatic nonmalignant perforations of the esophagus. Gastrointest Endosc 2003;58(3):356–61.

36. Gelbmann CM, Ratiu NL, Rath HC, et al. Use of self-expandable plastic stents for the treatment of esophageal perforations and symptomatic anastomotic leaks. Endoscopy 2004;36(8):695–9.

37. Johnsson E, Lundell L, Liedman B. Sealing of esophageal perforation or ruptures with expandable metallic stents: a prospective controlled study on treatment efficacy and limitations. Dis Esophagus 2005;18(4):262–6.

38. Fischer A, Thomusch O, Benz S, et al. Nonoperative treatment of 15 benign esophageal perforations with self-expandable covered metal stents. Ann Thorac Surg 2006;81(2):467–72.

39. Ott C, Ratiu N, Endlicher E, et al. Self-expanding Polyflex plastic stents in esophageal disease: various indications, complications, and outcomes. Surg Endosc 2007;21:889–96.

40. Freeman RK, Ascioti AJ, Wozniak TC. Postoperative esophageal leak management with the Polyflex esophageal stent. J Thorac Cardiovasc Surg 2007;133:333–8.

41. Tuebergen D, Rijcken E, Mennigen R, et al. Treatment of thoracic esophageal anastomotic leaks and esophageal perforations with endoluminal stents: efficacy and current limitations. J Gastrointest Surg 2008;12:1168–76.

42. Kim AW, Liptay MJ, Snow N, et al. Utility of silicone esophageal bypass stents in the management of delayed complex esophageal disruptions. Ann Thorac Surg 2008;85:1962–7.

43. Leers JM, Vivaldi C, Schafer H, et al. Endoscopic therapy for esophageal perforation or anastomotic leak with a self-expandable metallic stent. Surg Endosc 2009;23:2258–62.

44. Kiev J, Amendola M, Bouhaidar D, et al. A management algorithm for esophageal perforation. Am J Surg 2007;194(1):103–6.

45. Salminen P, Gullichsen R, Laine S. Use of self-expandable metal stents for the treatment of esophageal perforations and anastomotic leaks. Surg Endosc 2009;23(7):1526–30.

46. van Heel NC, Haringsma J, Spaander MC, et al. Short-term esophageal stenting in the management of benign perforations. Am J Gastroenterol 2010;105:1515–20.

47. Dai Y, Chopra S, Kneif S, et al. Management of esophageal anastomotic leaks, perforations, and fistulae with self-expanding plastic stents. J Thorac Cardiovasc Surg 2011;141(5):1213–7.

48. Dasari BV, Neely D, Kennedy A, et al. The role of esophageal stents in the management of esophageal anastomotic leaks and benign esophageal perforations. Ann Surg 2014;259(5):852–60.

49. Wahed S, Dent B, Jones R, et al. Spectrum of oesophageal perforations and their influence on management. Br J Surg 2014;101(1):e156–62.

50. Schorsch T, Muller C, Loske G. Endoscopic vacuum therapy of anastomotic leakage and iatrogenic perforation in the esophagus. Surg Endosc 2013;27(6):2040–5.
51. Modayil R, Friedel D, Stavropoulos SN. Endoscopic suture repair of a large mucosal perforation during peroral endoscopic myotomy for treatment of achalasia. Gastrointest Endosc 2014. [Epub ahead of print].
52. Li H, Linghu E, Wang X. Fibrin sealant for closure of mucosal penetration at the cardia during peroral endoscopic myotomy (POEM). Endoscopy 2012;44(Suppl 2 UCTN):E215–6. http://dx.doi.org/10.1055/s-0032-1309358.
53. Minami S, Gotoda T, Ono H, et al. Complete endoscopic closure of gastric perforation induced by endoscopic resection of early gastric cancer using endoclips can prevent surgery (with video). Gastrointest Endosc 2006;63(4):596–601.
54. Toyokawa T, Inaba T, Omote S, et al. Risk factors for perforation and delayed bleeding associated with endoscopic submucosal dissection for early gastric neoplasms: analysis of 1123 lesions. J Gastroenterol Hepatol 2012;27(5):907–12.
55. Tsunada S, Ogata S, Ohyama T, et al. Endoscopic closure of perforations caused by EMR in the stomach by application of metallic clips. Gastrointest Endosc 2003;57(7):948–51.
56. Fujishiro M, Yahagi N, Kakushima N, et al. Successful nonsurgical management of perforation complicating endoscopic submucosal dissection of gastrointestinal epithelial neoplasms. Endoscopy 2006;38(10):1001–6.
57. Imagawa A, Okada H, Kawahara Y, et al. Endoscopic submucosal dissection for early gastric cancer: results and degrees of technical difficulty as well as success. Endoscopy 2006;38(10):987–90.
58. Jeon SW, Jung MK, Kim SK, et al. Clinical outcomes for perforations during endoscopic submucosal dissection in patients with gastric lesions. Surg Endosc 2010;24(4):911–6. http://dx.doi.org/10.1007/s00464-009-0693-y.
59. Zhang Y, Wang X, Xiong G, et al. Complete defect closure of gastric submucosal tumors with purse-string sutures. Surg Endosc 2014;28(6):1844–51.
60. Zhang Y, Ye LP, Zhou XB, et al. Safety and efficacy of endoscopic excavation for gastric subepithelial tumors originating from the muscularis propria layer: results from a large study in China. J Clin Gastroenterol 2013;47(8):689–94. http://dx.doi.org/10.1097/MCG.0b013e3182908295.
61. Li L, Wang F, Wu B, et al. Endoscopic submucosal dissection of gastric fundus subepithelial tumors originating from the muscularis propria. Exp Ther Med 2013;6(2):391–5.
62. He Z, Sun C, Zheng Z, et al. Endoscopic submucosal dissection of large gastrointestinal stromal tumors in the esophagus and stomach. J Gastroenterol Hepatol 2013;28(2):262–7. http://dx.doi.org/10.1111/jgh.12056.
63. Zhou PH, Yao LQ, Qin XY, et al. Endoscopic full-thickness resection without laparoscopic assistance for gastric submucosal tumors originated from the muscularis propria. Surg Endosc 2011;25(9):2926–31. http://dx.doi.org/10.1007/s00464-011-1644-y.
64. Hookey LC, Khokhotva V, Bielawska B, et al. The Queen's closure: a novel technique for closure of endoscopic gastrotomy for natural orifice transluminal endoscopic surgery. Endoscopy 2009;41:149–53.
65. Hucl T, Benes M, Kocik M, et al. A novel double-endoloop technique for natural orifice transluminal endoscopic surgery gastric access site closure. Gastrointest Endosc 2010;71:806–11.
66. Ryska O, Martinek J, Dolezel R, et al. Feasibility of a novel single loop and clip gastrotomy closure (King's closure) after NOTES procedures in an experimental study. Gastroenterol Hepatol 2011;65:207–10.

67. Martínek J, Ryska O, Tuckova I, et al. Comparing over-the-scope clip versus endoloop and clips (KING closure) for access site closure: a randomized experimental study. Surg Endosc 2013;27:1203–10. http://dx.doi.org/10.1007/s00464-012-2576-x.

68. Hashiba K, Carvalho AM, Diniz G Jr, et al. Experimental endoscopic repair of gastric perforations with an omental patch and clips. Gastrointest Endosc 2001;54(4):500–4.

69. Zhang XL, Sun G, Tang P, et al. Endoscopic closure of experimental iatrogenic gastric fundus perforation using over-the-scope clips in a surviving canine model. J Gastroenterol Hepatol 2013;28(9):1502–6.

70. Singhal S, Atluri S, Changela K, et al. Endoscopic closure of gastric perforation using over-the-scope clip: a surgery-sparing approach. Gastrointest Endosc 2014;79(1):23.

71. Schlag C, Wilhelm D, von Delius S, et al. EndoResect study: endoscopic full-thickness resection of gastric subepithelial tumors. Endoscopy 2013;45(1): 4–11. http://dx.doi.org/10.1055/s-0032-1325760.

72. Gubler C, Bauerfeind P. Endoscopic closure of iatrogenic gastrointestinal tract perforations with the over-the-scope clip. Digestion 2012;85(4):302–7. http://dx.doi.org/10.1159/000336509.

73. Kantsevoy SV, Bitner M, Mitrakov AA, et al. Endoscopic suturing closure of large mucosal defects after endoscopic submucosal dissection is technically feasible, fast, and eliminates the need for hospitalization (with videos). Gastrointest Endosc 2014;79(3):503–7.

74. Song Y, Choi HS, Kim K, et al. A simple novel endoscopic successive suture device: a validation study for closure strength and reproducibility. Endoscopy 2013;45(8):655–60.

75. Han JH, Lee TH, Jung Y, et al. Rescue endoscopic band ligation of iatrogenic gastric perforations following failed endoclip closure. World J Gastroenterol 2013;19(6):955–9.

76. Sumiyama K, Gostout CJ. Clinical applications of submucosal endoscopy. Curr Opin Gastroenterol 2011;27(5):412–7.

77. Liu L, Chiu PW, Teoh AY, et al. Endoscopic suturing is superior to endoclips for closure of gastrotomy after natural orifices transluminal endoscopic surgery (NOTES): an ex vivo study. Surg Endosc 2014;28(4):1342–7.

78. Voermans RP, Worm AM, van Berge Henegouwen MI, et al. In vitro comparison and evaluation of seven gastric closure modalities for natural orifice transluminal endoscopic surgery (NOTES). Endoscopy 2008;40(7):595–601.

79. von Renteln D, Schmidt A, Vassiliou MC, et al. Natural orifice transluminal endoscopic surgery gastrotomy closure with an over-the-endoscope clip: a randomized, controlled porcine study (with videos). Gastrointest Endosc 2009; 70(4):732–9.

80. Bonin EA, Bingener J, Rajan E, et al. Omentum patch substitute for facilitating endoscopic repair of GI perforations: an early laparoscopic pilot study with a foam matrix plug (with video). Gastrointest Endosc 2013;77(1):123–30.

Closing Perforations and Postperforation Management in Endoscopy
Duodenal, Biliary, and Colorectal

Christine Boumitri, MD[a], Nikhil A. Kumta, MD[b], Milan Patel, MD[c], Michel Kahaleh, MD, FASGE[b],*

KEYWORDS

- Endoscopy • Perforation • Closure • Surgery • Interventional radiology
- Endoscopic retrograde cholangiopancreatography • Through-the-scope clips
- Over-the-scope clips

KEY POINTS

- Early recognition of perforation is essential.
- Some cases can be managed conservatively or endoscopically.
- Endoscopic closure can be successful.
- Recognizing emergencies after perforations is mandatory for immediate action.
- Surgical consultation is essential.
- Patients who fail endoscopic closure should elect to undergo surgery.
- Multiple endoscopic closure devices are available.

INTRODUCTION

With the evolution of endoscopy, the increased use of novel and innovative therapeutic endoscopic procedures has been associated with a simultaneous increase in the rate of associated adverse events. Gastrointestinal perforations, fistulas, and anastomotic leakages are not limited to endoscopic procedures but can also be the result of laparoscopic surgeries. Iatrogenic luminal perforations carry a significant morbidity and mortality, and can necessitate surgical interventions if not recognized early on.

[a] Department of Medicine, Staten Island University Hospital, 475 Seaview Avenue, Staten Island, NY 10305, USA; [b] Division of Gastroenterology and Hepatology, Weill Cornell Medical College, 1305 York Avenue, 4th Floor, New York, NY 10021, USA; [c] Division of Gastroenterology, Robert Wood Johnson Medical School, 501 Fellowship Road, Mount Laurel, NJ 08054, USA
* Corresponding author. Division of Gastroenterology and Hepatology, Weill Cornell Medical College, 1305 York Avenue, 4th Floor, New York, NY 10021.
E-mail address: mkahaleh@gmail.com

Gastrointest Endoscopy Clin N Am 25 (2015) 47–54
http://dx.doi.org/10.1016/j.giec.2014.09.010
1052-5157/15/$ – see front matter © 2015 Elsevier Inc. All rights reserved.
giendo.theclinics.com

The development of natural orifice transluminal endoscopic surgery (NOTES), whereby hollow visceral perforation is intentionally performed to enter the abdominal cavity, marked a footprint in the endoscopic nonsurgical management of gastrointestinal perforations.[1] Endoscopic closure of perforations can be successfully achieved using a variety of devices. Recently, Baron and colleagues[2] described the "Ten Commandments of endoscopic perforations" (**Box 1**) in which the emphasis is on early recognition of postprocedural perforations and adequate management of its complications. Intervening early on to close these perforations may result in a better outcome. Recognizing conditions that require emergent action such as tension pneumothorax, abdominal compartment syndrome, and peritonitis are crucial in preventing mortality.

CLOSURE OF PERFORATIONS
Duodenal Perforations

Duodenal perforations can be divided into 2 types, periampullary and nonperiampullary, with the first being most commonly associated with therapeutic endoscopic retrograde cholangiopancreatography (ERCP). The use of the side-viewing duodenoscope confers a higher risk of perforation because direct view of the tract being intubated with the scope cannot be achieved. This risk increases when surgical diversions such a Billroth II gastrectomy exist.

Periampullary perforations

Perforation can occur in 0.3% to 1% of ERCPs.[1] Risk factors include sphincterotomy, sphincter of Oddi dysfunction, and dilated common bile duct.[3] Elderly patients tend to have periampullary diverticulum, which can increase the risk of perforations not only by making cannulation more difficult but also by distorting anatomic landmarks used to perform sphincterotomy. Periampullary perforations can be divided into 4 subgroups according to Stapfer and colleagues.[4]

Type I corresponds to lateral or medial duodenal wall perforations, type II peri-Vaterian injury, type III bile or pancreatic duct injury, and type IV the presence of retroperitoneal air alone.[4]

Box 1
The Ten Commandments of endoscopic perforations

1. Prompt recognition of endoscopic perforation is essential to improvement in outcome

2. The presence of extraluminal air does not automatically mean the need for surgery

3. The volume of extraluminal air is not necessarily proportional to the size of the perforation

4. Extraluminal air per se is not infectious

5. Extraluminal air under pressure is a medical emergency

6. Extraluminal air can dissect into distant spaces

7. Residual extraluminal air may persist without clinical significance

8. Perforations tend to close after drainage or diversion of luminal contents

9. Free oral or injected contrast material extravasation should elicit prompt intervention

10. Failed endoscopic closure of a perforation generally requires surgical intervention

From Baron TH, Wong Kee Song LM, Zielinski MD, et al. A comprehensive approach to the management of acute endoscopic perforations. Gastrointest Endosc 2012;76(4):838–59; with permission from Elsevier.

Type I lesions are the result of a countercoup injury with the tip of the scope; they are large and usually require surgical correction with an omental patch, pyloric exclusion, gastrojejunostomy, or other surgical intervention. However, there have been successful cases of endoscopic closure using endoclips or over-the-scope (OTS) clips when the size is less than 15 mm.[5,6] Clipping using through-the-scope (TTS) mucosal clips can be achieved by placing multiple clips in a linear fashion when the perforation is small and accessible, or with the aid of a transparent cap to suction tissue when angulation is present.[5,7] Medial wall perforations are more difficult to close endoscopically because of their anatomic location and the risk of clipping the ampulla.

Management of type II injuries is less clear. Treatment is possible using a biliary stent or a TTS clip in addition to the use of a nasoduodenal drain to divert pancreatic and biliary secretions, which are toxic and can lead to clinical decompensation. However, 10% to 43% of patients will require surgical intervention.[4,8,9]

Type III perforations are generally easy to treat.[10] Bile duct perforations can be managed by a plastic stent or temporary placement of fully covered self-expandable metal stents (FCSEMS).[11]

Type IV perforations are usually managed conservatively with no surgical intervention, even when large extravasation of air exists in the absence of tension pneumoperitoneum.[12] Pneumoperitoneum can be present in up to 29% of asymptomatic patients who undergo uncomplicated interventions.[13]

Nonperiampullary perforations

Duodenal perforations that are not periampullary are the result of direct trauma to the duodenum from the endoscope or the result of therapeutic interventions such as polypectomies or stricture dilations. Similar to type I perforations, they are mostly managed surgically because of the anatomic difficulty for endoscopic clip deployment. However, TTS clips and OTS clips have been deployed successfully in humans.[14] The use of the FCSEMS is another available option. If retroperitoneal collections develop they can be drained by Interventional radiologists. If blood clots are seen in the drainage catheters the clinician should be suspicious for development of vascular complications such as pseudoaneuvrysms. When hemodynamic instability occurs or endoscopic and interventional radiologic procedures fail, surgical exploration is required.

Biliary Tract Perforations

Biliary tract perforations are the result of wire manipulation, especially in the setting of a stricture whereby repetitive attempts to bypass it are needed. Early recognition is necessary, and endoscopic treatment by placing a stent over the perforation is successful. Some patients can be managed conservatively with intravenous antibiotics when the perforation is below the stricture level. Biliary collections into the peritoneum can be managed by percutaneous or endoscopic drainage. If endoscopy fails to treat the perforation, percutaneous biliary drainage above the level of perforation is an alternative. If surgery is required, transfer to a tertiary care surgical center where expert surgeons are available is needed.[2]

Colorectal Perforations

Colonoscopy is complicated by perforation in 0.01% to 0.3% of cases.[2,15] The incidence increases during therapeutic interventions, and was reported to be 1.2% during snare polypectomy and 5% during endoscopic submucosal dissection (ESD).[15] Management of these perforations depends on the location of the perforation. In particular, whether a perforation is colonic or rectal dictates a different management approach.

Colonic perforations

Colonic perforations related to diagnostic colonoscopy are typically due to mechanical trauma secondary to impaction of the endoscope tip, or antimesenteric impaction of the endoscope body against the colonic wall. The sigmoid colon is the most common site of colon perforation owing to its tortuous nature and frequent presence of diverticula, pedunculated polyps, and postoperative adhesions in this region. The rate of perforation in the rectosigmoid colon was reported to be 65%.[16] The descending and ascending colon is the site of perforation in 15% and 8% of cases, respectively.[16] Another area where perforations tend to occur is the cecum. Cecal perforations are induced by barotrauma, typically present in a difficult colonoscopy with overinflation. Perforation rates in the ascending colon and rectum are reported to be equal to that of the cecum, at 4%.[16]

These perforations remain unrecognized until pneumoperitoneum develops. When it occurs, needle decompression should be performed to eliminate tension pneumoperitoneum. Further management depends on the clinical status of the patient, the size of the perforation, the presence of extraluminal fecal soiling, the degree of colon preparation, and the time elapsed after the perforation.[15] When the perforation is recognized during or immediately after the procedure, closing with TTS clips or OTS clips should be attempted when the perforation is less than 2 cm. Band ligation can also be useful for closing colon perforations that fail placement of TTS mucosal clips.[15,17–19] It is recommended to close vertical perforations from the top down and horizontal/circular perforations from left to right.[15]

A new innovative approach to close colonic perforations, termed the tulip bundle technique, has been described, which requires an endoloop, TTS clips, and glue. Clips are positioned on the perforation edges, followed by tightening of the defect with an endoloop and applying glue to their bases to complete the closure.[15]

Colonic perforations related to therapeutic colonoscopic interventions differ in mechanism from those caused by diagnostic colonoscopy. More frequently localized to the cecum and right-side colon, transmural electrocautery injury is the leading cause of perforation. For example, during polypectomy the identification of a target sign on the excision site and on the specimen indicates perforation, and should be closed endoscopically immediately.[17]

It is very important to monitor patients closely for any deterioration that would require surgical intervention. Abdominal computed tomography (CT) with rectal contrast can help identify continuous leakage. If a collection is identified, it should be drained. When colonic perforations open into the peritoneal space, surgical exploration with washout and fecal diversion is recommended. Perforations isolated to the extraperitoneal space generally can be treated nonoperatively.

Rectal perforations

Causes of rectal perforation include endoscope retroflexion, endoscopic mucosal resection, and ESD. Rectal perforation is diagnosed by direct or radiographic visualization of evidence of unintended penetration beyond the rectal mucosa. Typically these perforations are moderate, and lead to subcutaneous emphysema that is treated by nothing per mouth and broad-spectrum antibiotics. These emphysemas usually resolve in a matter of days. Defect closure using TTS clips and OTS clips can be effective.[18–22]

POSTPERFORATION MANAGEMENT

Iatrogenic perforations are serious adverse events that can carry high morbidity and mortality, especially when more worrisome complications develop. **Table 1** lists the

Table 1
Suggested management of some adverse events encountered with endoscopy

Adverse Event	Management
1. Mediastinitis	Nil per mouth, intravenous hydration, intravenous antibiotics, surgical evaluation for possible debridement/collection drainage/closing perforation
2. Peritonitis	Nil per mouth, intravenous hydration, intravenous antibiotics, surgical evaluation for possible lavage/collection drainage/closing perforation
3. Subcutaneous emphysema	Usually resolves spontaneously in few days. Massive air tracking into soft tissues of the neck can result in airway obstruction and may require endotracheal intubation
4. Tension pneumothorax	Immediate needle decompression of the affected site with a needle catheter inserted along the midclavicular line in the second intercostal space followed by chest tube insertion
5. Tension pneumoperitoneum	Immediate decompression with an 18- or 20-gauge needle into the abdomen with the patient in the supine position

suggested management of a few endoscopic adverse events that may be encountered.

In duodenal perforations, close monitoring is required with CT imaging, surgical consultation, and a repeat CT scan at 48 hours to follow progression and especially to look for fluid collections requiring drainage. Antibiotics, fasting, nasogastric suctioning, and proton-pump inhibitors (PPI) are the mainstay of postoperative care. Oral intake can be resumed after the fourth day if no further leakage is identified.[23]

In colonic perforation, the postoperative management remains similar to that for other sites of perforation. There are risk factors that predict unfavorable clinical outcome in the first 24 hours, including severe abdominal pain, large perforations, leukocytosis, high temperature, and tension pneumoperitoneum (**Box 2**).[24,25] The use of carbon dioxide (CO_2) remains important in all gastrointestinal perforations because it is associated with less peritoneal irritation and helps maintain hemodynamic stability because it is more rapidly absorbed than air.

OUTCOMES

The outcomes of endoscopic closure depend on the acuity and etiology of gastrointestinal perforations (iatrogenic, anastomotic leak, fistula, and so forth). In an article elsewhere in this issue, Dr. Stavropoulos and colleagues review perforation closure

---

Box 2
Risk factors associated with unfavorable outcome 24 hours after colonic perforations

Severe abdominal pain requiring narcotic analgesics

Perforation resulting from diagnostic colonoscopy or larger than 10 mm

Leukocytosis greater than 10,000 mm^3

Temperature 37°C or higher

Large pneumoperitoneum ($\geq$3 cm between the upper liver margin and the right diaphragm on plain chest radiograph)

of the esophagus and stomach, there is a more detailed review of the existing literature regarding outcomes using TTS mucosal clips, suturing devices, and covered stents.

The technical success rate of TTS mucosal clip closure ranges between 59% and 100% of cases.[26,27] Drawbacks associated with the use of TTS clips include early detachment, minor leaks secondary to inadequate sealing, increased risk of pneumoperitoneum owing to longer procedure time, and longer insufflation.[17,28] The latter can be decreased by the use of CO_2 instead of air.[29]

The technical success rate of OTS clips has been reported to be 91% to 93%, with a clinical success of 89%.[30,31] As previously mentioned, these clips have been successfully used to close esophageal, gastric, small intestinal, and colonic perforations. Despite providing a full-thickness closure, the OTS clip has the disadvantage of having to completely withdraw the scope to mount the device on the outside of the endoscope. The use of a twin grasper with independently movable arms can be also technically challenging, especially when the perforation edges are everted.[32,33]

There are limited published data regarding the success and outcome of using endoscopic suturing devices to close perforations. However, the use of suturing has been increasing. Its use for closing mucosal defects after ESD has been reported to be feasible and efficient, with decreased need for hospitalization.[34]

Covered stents have been used to bypass perforations, thus preventing any further leak. However, they are associated with a high rate of migration reaching up to 30%, and should be replaced after 8 weeks.[35] Various techniques of stent anchoring (suturing, clipping, and so forth) have been described to decrease stent migration rates.[36,37]

SUMMARY

Novel endoluminal surgical techniques in addition to the advent of improved endoscopic devices to close perforations has heralded a new and exciting era, pushing the boundaries of endoscopic surgery. With these advancements it is paramount to be able to manage patients with perforations appropriately. However, most of the available data regarding endoscopic closure are based on case reports, small retrospective series, small pilot studies, and prospective studies conducted on animals. Therefore, management depends on the overall clinical scenario in addition to the size and location of the perforation and the timing of recognition. If a defect is noticed during an endoscopic procedure and is amenable to endoscopic closure, it should be closed immediately. Rapid endoscopic closure of perforations may eliminate the need for surgical intervention and its associated morbidity and mortality. Closure can be achieved by a variety of methods and devices, as described herein. If a perforation is detected postprocedure, recognition is key to a good clinical outcome. Delay in recognition and closure of perforations can lead to clinical deterioration and a worse outcome for the patient.

REFERENCES

1. Volgyi Z, Szenes M, Gasztonyi B. Az endoszkopos retrograd cholangiopancreatographia soran kialakult perforaciok tipusai es kezelesuk. [Types and management of perforations occurring during endoscopic retrograde cholangiopancreatography]. Orv Hetil 2014;155(7):248–54 [in Hungarian].
2. Baron TH, Wong Kee Song LM, Zielinski MD, et al. A comprehensive approach to the management of acute endoscopic perforations (with videos). Gastrointest Endosc 2012;76(4):838–59.
3. Enns R, Eloubeidi MA, Mergener K, et al. ERCP-related perforations: risk factors and management. Endoscopy 2002;34(4):293–8.

4. Stapfer M, Selby RR, Stain SC, et al. Management of duodenal perforation after endoscopic retrograde cholangiopancreatography and sphincterotomy. Ann Surg 2000;232(2):191–8.
5. Knudson K, Raeburn CD, McIntyre RC Jr, et al. Management of duodenal and pancreaticobiliary perforations associated with periampullary endoscopic procedures. Am J Surg 2008;196(6):975–81 [discussion: 981–2].
6. Parodi A, Repici A, Pedroni A, et al. Endoscopic management of GI perforations with a new over-the-scope clip device (with videos). Gastrointest Endosc 2010; 72(4):881–6.
7. Al Ghossaini N, Lucidarme D, Bulois P. Endoscopic treatment of iatrogenic gastrointestinal perforations: an overview. Dig Liver Dis 2014;46(3):195–203.
8. Kim JH, Yoo BM, Kim JH, et al. Management of ERCP-related perforations: outcomes of single institution in Korea. J Gastrointest Surg 2009;13(4):728–34.
9. Kayhan B, Akdogan M, Sahin B. ERCP subsequent to retroperitoneal perforation caused by endoscopic sphincterotomy. Gastrointest Endosc 2004;60(5):833–5.
10. The Bakke case. Hosp Pract 1978;13(2):17.
11. Jeon HJ, Han JH, Park S, et al. Endoscopic sphincterotomy-related perforation in the common bile duct successfully treated by placement of a covered metal stent. Endoscopy 2011;43(Suppl 2 UCTN):E295–6.
12. Ferrara F, Luigiano C, Billi P, et al. Pneumothorax, pneumomediastinum, pneumoperitoneum, pneumoretroperitoneum, and subcutaneous emphysema after ERCP. Gastrointest Endosc 2009;69(7):1398–401.
13. Genzlinger JL, McPhee MS, Fisher JK, et al. Significance of retroperitoneal air after endoscopic retrograde cholangiopancreatography with sphincterotomy. Am J Gastroenterol 1999;94(5):1267–70.
14. Haider S, Kahaleh M. The use of endoscopic clipping devices in the treatment of iatrogenic duodenal perforation. Gastroenterol Hepatol 2010;6(10):660–1.
15. Raju GS, Saito Y, Matsuda T, et al. Endoscopic management of colonoscopic perforations (with videos). Gastrointest Endosc 2011;74(6):1380–8.
16. Tam MS, Abbas MA. Perforation following colorectal endoscopy: what happens beyond the endoscopy suite? Perm J 2013;17(2):17–21.
17. Cho SB, Lee WS, Joo YE, et al. Therapeutic options for iatrogenic colon perforation: feasibility of endoscopic clip closure and predictors of the need for early surgery. Surg Endosc 2012;26(2):473–9.
18. Seebach L, Bauerfeind P, Gubler C, et al. Therapeutic options for over-the-scope clips for gastrointestinal perforation. Endoscopy 2010;42(12):1108–11.
19. Han JH, Park S, Youn S. Endoscopic closure of colon perforation with band ligation; salvage technique after endoclip failure. Clin Gastroenterol Hepatol 2011; 9(6):e54–5.
20. Mocciaro F, Curcio G, Tarantino I, et al. Tulip bundle technique and fibrin glue injection: unusual treatment of colonic perforation. World J Gastroenterol 2011; 17(8):1088–90.
21. Swan MP, Bourke MJ, Moss A, et al. The target sign: an endoscopic marker for the resection of the muscularis propria and potential perforation during colonic endoscopic mucosal resection. Gastrointest Endosc 2011;73(1):79–85.
22. Ahlawat SK, Charabaty A, Benjamin S. Rectal perforation caused by retroflexion maneuver during colonoscopy: closure with endoscopic clips. Gastrointest Endosc 2008;67(4):771–3.
23. Katsinelos P, Kountouras J, Chatzimavroudis G, et al. Endoscopic closure of a large iatrogenic rectal perforation using endoloop/clips technique. Acta Gastroenterol Belg 2008;72(3):357–9.

24. Coriat R, Leblanc S, Pommaret E, et al. Endoscopic management of endoscopic submucosal dissection perforations: a new over-the-scope clip device. Gastrointest Endosc 2011;73(5):1067–9.
25. Eroglu A, Turkyilmaz A, Aydin Y, et al. Current management of esophageal perforation: 20 years experience. Dis Esophagus 2009;22(4):374–80.
26. D'Cunha J, Rueth NM, Groth SS, et al. Esophageal stents for anastomotic leaks and perforations. J Thorac Cardiovasc Surg 2011;142(1):39–46.e1.
27. Kim BS, Kim IG, Ryu BY, et al. Management of endoscopic retrograde cholangiopancreatography-related perforations. J Korean Surg Soc 2011;81(3): 195–204.
28. Fujishiro M, Yahagi N, Kakushima N, et al. Successful nonsurgical management of perforation complicating endoscopic submucosal dissection of gastrointestinal epithelial neoplasms. Endoscopy 2006;38(10):1001–6.
29. Magdeburg R, Collet P, Post S, et al. Endoclipping of iatrogenic colonic perforation to avoid surgery. Surg Endosc 2008;22(6):1500–4.
30. Diez-Redondo P, Blanco JI, Lorenzo-Pelayo S, et al. A novel system for endoscopic closure of iatrogenic colon perforations using the Ovesco(R) clip and omental patch. Rev Esp Enferm Dig 2012;104(10):550–2.
31. Minami S, Gotoda T, Ono H, et al. Complete endoscopic closure of gastric perforation induced by endoscopic resection of early gastric cancer using endoclips can prevent surgery (with video). Gastrointest Endosc 2006;63(4):596–601.
32. Gubler C, Bauerfeind P. Endoscopic closure of iatrogenic gastrointestinal tract perforations with the over-the-scope clip. Digestion 2012;85(4):302–7.
33. Junquera F, Martinez-Bauer E, Miquel M, et al. OVESCO: un sistema prometedor de cierre endoscopico de las perforaciones del tracto digestivo. [OVESCO: a promising system for endoscopic closure of gastrointestinal tract perforations]. Gastroenterol Hepatol 2011;34(8):568–72 [in Spanish].
34. Kantsevoy SV, Bitner M, Mitrakov AA, et al. Endoscopic suturing closure of large mucosal defects after endoscopic submucosal dissection is technically feasible, fast, and eliminates the need for hospitalization (with videos). Gastrointest Endosc 2014;79(3):503–7.
35. Motta G, Facchini GM, D'Auria E. Objective conditioned-reflex audiometry in children. Acta Otolaryngol Suppl 1970;273:1–49.
36. Song HY, Jung HY, Park SI, et al. Covered retrievable expandable nitinol stents in patients with benign esophageal strictures: initial experience. Radiology 2000; 217(2):551–7.
37. Vanbiervliet G, Filippi J, Karimdjee BS, et al. The role of clips in preventing migration of fully covered metallic esophageal stents: a pilot comparative study. Surg Endosc 2012;26(1):53–9.

Adverse Events Related to Colonic Endoscopic Mucosal Resection and Polypectomy

 CrossMark

Amrita Sethi, MD[a],*, Louis M. Wong Kee Song, MD[b]

KEYWORDS

- Adverse events ● Endoscopic closure ● Endoscopic hemostasis
- Endoscopic mucosal resection ● Perforation ● Polypectomy
- Postpolypectomy bleeding ● Postpolypectomy syndrome

KEY POINTS

- Adverse events from endoscopic mucosal resection (EMR) and polypectomy include immediate and delayed bleeding, perforation, and postpolypectomy syndrome.
- Intraprocedural bleeding can be managed effectively with a variety of endoscopic modalities, including clips, detachable snares, and contact thermal probes or graspers, with or without epinephrine injection; the selection of one or a combination of techniques depends on the type of lesion, completeness of resection, device availability, and operator preference.
- Delayed postpolypectomy bleeding is self-limited in most cases and can be managed conservatively; endoscopic hemostasis is reserved for recurrent or ongoing bleeding.
- Immediate recognition and closure of EMR- or polypectomy-induced perforations are key determinants for a successful outcome. Endoscopic versus surgical management of perforations depends on defect size and access, presence of extraluminal contamination, and clinical status of the patient.
- Mucosal clip placement constitutes the mainstay of endoscopic therapy for perforation, although newer devices, such as the over-the-scope clip and endoscopic suturing, have expanded the options for closure.
- Close monitoring post perforation closure is essential in the context of a multidisciplinary approach, with prompt surgical intervention in the presence of clinical deterioration.
- Postpolypectomy syndrome is a transmural thermal injury that can mimic perforation, but whose prognosis is excellent with conservative management.

[a] Division of Digestive and Liver Diseases, Columbia University, 161 Fort Washington Avenue, Herbert Irving Pavilion, Suite 862, New York, NY 10032, USA; [b] Division of Gastroenterology and Hepatology, Mayo Clinic, 200 1st Street Southwest, Rochester, MN 55905, USA
* Corresponding author.
E-mail address: asethimd@gmail.com

Gastrointest Endoscopy Clin N Am 25 (2015) 55–69
http://dx.doi.org/10.1016/j.giec.2014.09.007

Videos demonstrating the prevention and management of adverse events associated with polypectomy and endoscopic mucosal resection of colonic lesions accompany this article at http://www.giendo.theclinics.com/

INTRODUCTION

Colonoscopy is a commonly performed procedure. The rate of adverse events (AEs) is 2.8 per 1000 screening colonoscopies.[1] These AEs include cardiovascular and pulmonary events, abdominal pain, hemorrhage, perforation, postpolypectomy syndrome (PPS), infection, and death. Serious AEs, such as hemorrhage and perforation, occur most frequently when colonoscopy is performed with polypectomy.[1] This article highlights the prevention and management of AEs associated with polypectomy and endoscopic mucosal resection (EMR) of colonic lesions.

POLYPECTOMY AND ENDOSCOPIC MUCOSAL RESECTION OF COLONIC LESIONS

Standard polypectomy techniques involve hot or cold snaring without submucosal fluid injection. Lesions that are less than or equal to 1 cm in size can be resected safely via cold snare, whereas hot snare is usually used for larger lesions. A blended current is commonly used during hot snare polypectomy; however, there are proponents for the use of pure coagulation current.[2]

The use of hot biopsy forceps is not recommended because of increased risk of complications, such as PPS and delayed perforation, and the availability of safer polypectomy techniques.[2]

EMR is a modified version of saline-assisted polypectomy that is used in the colon to facilitate lesion resection and mitigate the risk of perforation associated with the removal of large sessile polyps. Although technical variations exist, most EMR techniques are centered on the concept of injecting a solution to provide a cushion between the mucosal and deeper layers of the colon wall. Specialized band ligation and cap-assisted EMR devices are commonly used in the esophagus and stomach, but have limited applicability in the colon. EMR in the colon usually consists of freehand snare resection following submucosal fluid injection. En bloc snare resection is preferred so that the depth and lateral margins of the resected specimen can be accurately assessed at histopathology, and this is generally feasible if the lesion is less than 2 cm in size. For lesions that are 2 cm or larger, piecemeal resection is recommended to decrease the risk of perforation.

The submucosal lift can be performed using a variety of solutions (**Table 1**). A commonly used injectate consists of saline stained with a few drops of a dye (indigo carmine or methylene blue), with or without dilute epinephrine. A post-EMR defect that

Table 1 Selected solutions used for submucosal injection			
Solution	Cushion Duration	Cost	Tissue Damage
Saline	+	Cheap	No
Hypertonic saline	++	Cheap	Yes
50% Dextrose	++	Cheap	Yes
Glycerol	++	—	No
Hyaluronic acid	+++	Expensive	No
Hydroxypropyl methylcellulose	+++	Cheap	No

uniformly stains blue confirms that the resection plane is limited to the submucosal layer (**Fig. 1**). A wide range of dilute epinephrine (1:10,000–1:100,000) in the mixture has been reported. Although epinephrine minimizes the risk of immediate bleeding and facilitates endoscopic visualization by maintaining a dry resection field, it does not prevent delayed bleeding.[3,4] A longer-lasting fluid cushion can be obtained with the use of viscous solutions, such as hetastarch, succinylated gelatin, and hydroxypropyl methylcellulose. These solutions may reduce procedural time and the number of resections needed for completing piecemeal EMR.[5]

ADVERSE EVENTS OF ENDOSCOPIC MUCOSAL RESECTION AND POLYPECTOMY

The major AEs related to EMR and polypectomy include hemorrhage, perforation, and PPS. Clinically relevant stricture formation can result from wide or circumferential EMR, but this is more of an issue in the esophagus than in the colon.

Hemorrhage

Hemorrhage is the most common AE of colonoscopy with polypectomy,[6–8] with reported incidences ranging from 0.1% to 0.5% for clinically significant bleeding.[9] Hemorrhage can occur at the time of the procedure (immediate bleeding) or hours to weeks (delayed bleeding) after the procedure.[10] However, most delayed bleeding events occur within 2 weeks. Intraprocedural and delayed bleeding caused by EMR of large

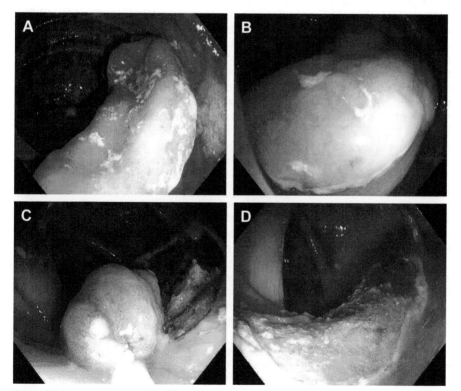

Fig. 1. (A) Large serrated polyp. (B) Submucosal fluid injection with methylene blue solution and dilute epinephrine. (C) Piecemeal EMR. (D) Uniform blue stain of the submucosal defect.

colorectal lesions occur in 1% to 11% of cases, although a wide range of EMR-related bleeding estimates have been reported (0%–45%).[11,12]

Predictors of hemorrhage

Several factors related to the patient, lesion, and resection technique can predict the risk of hemorrhage following polypectomy and EMR. In a large prospective study involving 9336 polypectomies in 5152 patients, immediate postpolypectomy bleeding occurred in 4% of cases. Significant risk factors for immediate bleeding included age 65 and older, use of anticoagulants, comorbid cardiovascular or chronic renal disease, polyp size greater than 1 cm, lesions featuring pedunculated polyps or laterally spreading tumors, suboptimal bowel preparation, and use of cutting current.[13] In another study involving 6617 polypectomies in 3138 patients, delayed postpolypectomy bleeding occurred in 38 (0.57%) lesions and 37 (1.2%) patients. Hypertension and polyp size (10.0 ± 6.9 vs 5.6 ± 3.8 mm; P<.0001) were associated with increased risk of delayed bleeding, whereas lesion location and resection method did not seem to affect the bleeding risk.[10] Other studies, however, have shown an increased risk for bleeding following removal of right-sided colonic lesions. In one small case-control study, polyp location and size were found to be independent risk factors for delayed bleeding. Polyps located in the right colon had an odds ratio (OR) of 4.67 (95% confidence interval [CI], 1.88–11.61; P = .001) for delayed hemorrhage.[14] Similarly, polyp location proximal to the splenic flexure (OR, 2.9; 95% CI, 1.05–8.1) and size (OR, 1.3; 95% CI, 1.1–1.7 for each 10 mm increase in size) were associated with delayed bleeding in another report of colonic EMR for large (≥2 cm) lesions.[15]

In a study involving 1657 patients and a polypectomy-related bleeding rate of 2.2%, warfarin was found to be an independent risk factor (OR, 13.37; 95% CI, 4.20–43.65) for polypectomy-induced bleeding, but not the use of nonsteroidal anti-inflammatory drugs, aspirin, and other antiplatelet agents.[16] Data on the use of uninterrupted clopidogrel and postpolypectomy bleeding are conflicting. In a recent meta-analysis, continued clopidogrel use was shown to increase the risk of delayed but not immediate postpolypectomy bleeding, with a pooled relative risk ratio of 4.66 (95% CI, 2.37–9.17; P<.01).[17] In contrast, a case-control study demonstrated no significant differences in the rates of delayed bleeding among clopidogrel users and nonusers, although the study findings were mostly applicable to small polyps (<1 cm).[18]

There is no standardization regarding the use of electrosurgical current during snare polypectomy, and evidence-based data on which to base the optimal setting for EMR and polypectomy are lacking. In one study, all immediate postpolypectomy bleeding occurred when a blended current was used, whereas all delayed postpolypectomy bleeding occurred with the use of coagulation current.[19] In a recent study, clinically significant delayed postpolypectomy hemorrhage was associated with the use of an electrosurgical current not controlled by a microprocessor (OR, 2.03; P = .038).[12]

In summary, several variables have been associated with the risk for postpolypectomy bleeding. Risk factors that seem to be consistent among studies include polyp size greater than 1 to 2 cm, flat or laterally spreading lesions and pedunculated polyps with thick stalks, right-sided colonic lesions, resection technique (including type of electrosurgical current utilized), and coagulation status.

Management of postpolypectomy hemorrhage

Immediate (intraprocedural) hemorrhage Constricting the residual stump with the snare and holding pressure can usually control immediate bleeding following transection of a pedunculated polyp with a thick stalk. If significant bleeding recurs following snare loosening, reconstricting the stalk for an additional period of time may result in hemostasis or, alternatively, dilute epinephrine (1:10,000 solution) can be injected in the base of the stump to reduce or stop bleeding and enable clearing of the field of view for more definitive therapy, such as placement of clips, a detachable snare (endoloop), or direct suture ligation.

In the situation where the residual stalk is too short to grasp with the electrosurgical snare or an endoloop, several hemostatic measures can be used, alone or in combination. Dilute epinephrine can be injected in and around the bleeding point, but care should be undertaken to avoid overinjection on the aboral side to avoid lifting the lesion away from view and placing it in a difficult position for subsequent therapy. The use of epinephrine is only a temporary measure and this should be followed by more definitive therapy. When technically feasible, the application of mechanical hemostatic devices is preferable because they do not extend the depth of tissue injury, which occurs with the use of thermal devices. Endoscopic clips can be placed directly on the bleeding point or on the residual stalk. Alternatively, a detachable snare can be used if access to and length of the residual stalk are favorable. If thermal probes are used, coaptive coagulation for 3 to 5 seconds is recommended at settings of 15 J for the heater probe and 12 to 15 W for the bipolar coagulation probe. The tip of the snare can also be used to control bleeding, but caution using this technique is warranted to avoid deep monopolar thermal injury. The Coagrasper device (Olympus Corp., Tokyo, Japan) is a monopolar coagulation forceps designed for grasping, tenting, and sealing of nonbleeding and bleeding vessels. Although it is used primarily during endoscopic submucosal dissection (ESD) for coagulation of submucosal vessels, it can be effective at grasping and sealing the bleeding vessel atop the resected stalk or polypectomy base, provided the grasped tissue can be tented.

Treatment of bleeding that occurs during en bloc or piecemeal EMR may not be necessary (eg, mild transient oozing at the resection edge). Endoscopic therapy should be reserved for active bleeding that interferes with completion of the procedure, or persistent oozing that has not ceased by the end of the procedure. An endoscope with forward water jet irrigation is helpful to precisely identify the location of the bleeding point. An actively bleeding vessel within an EMR defect is best treated with the grasping coagulation forceps (Coagrasper) using a soft coagulation mode at a power setting that produces prompt tissue coagulation (this can vary depending on the power setting [30–60 W] and type of electrosurgical unit; Video 1) or with clip placement (**Fig. 2**), with or without prior epinephrine injection. Clip placement, however,

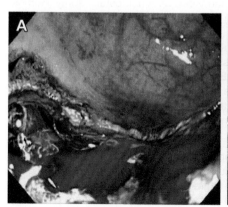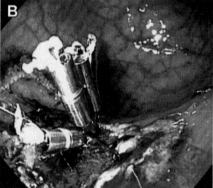

Fig. 2. (*A*) Active bleeding following en bloc EMR of rectal polyp. (*B*) Hemostasis achieved following clip placement.

should be avoided if it has the potential to interfere with completion of resection. Argon plasma coagulation and contact thermal probes can extend the depth of tissue injury and should be used with caution.

Delayed hemorrhage In the setting of delayed postpolypectomy hemorrhage, the basic tenets regarding management of gastrointestinal (GI) bleeding should be followed, including triage to the appropriate service (ward or intensive care unit) based on the severity of bleeding and patient comorbidities, fluid and blood transfusions as appropriate, withholding anticoagulation and antiplatelet agents, and correction of coagulopathy if present.

Patients in whom bloody bowel movements have ceased at the time of admission can usually be managed conservatively because rebleeding is uncommon. If there are no signs of ongoing bleeding during administration of the colon preparation, colonoscopy may be deferred with the exception of patients requiring prompt resumption of antithrombotic therapy. In patients in whom bleeding recurs during observation or in those with ongoing bloody stools, urgent colonoscopy should be performed.

The significance and rebleeding rates of stigmata of recent hemorrhage found in postpolypectomy ulcer beds are not as well studied as those related to bleeding peptic ulcers. In general, the ulcer experience is translatable to the postpolypectomy ulcer. Postpolypectomy ulcers with clean bases or flat, pigmented spots do not require intervention. Pigmented protuberances (visible vessels), adherent clots, and active bleeding require endoscopic therapy. Clip placement or thermal therapy, alone or in combination with epinephrine injection, can be used to treat the underlying bleeding stigmata. Mucosal clips can be applied directly on the vessel or the entire postpolypectomy defect (Video 2). The latter may not be possible because of induration of the polypectomy base margins (Video 3). Similarly, it may be difficult for the Coagrasper device to grasp and tent a visible vessel within the indurated ulcer bed. This can result in avulsion of the vessel with subsequent bleeding. Some of these lesions may be amenable to placement of an over-the-scope clip (OTSC; Ovesco Endoscopy AG, Tübingen, Germany) (Video 4), but practical issues may limit the use of this device because removal of the endoscope is required for loading of the OTSC. Similarly, direct suture ligation may be performed after withdrawing the colonoscope (OverStitch; Apollo Endosurgery, Austin, TX), provided the bleeding site can be reached with a double-channel upper endoscope. An indurated polypectomy base provides a safety cushion for the use of contact thermal probes. These modalities may be more effective in this setting (see Video 3). A hemostatic spray (Hemospray; Cook Medical Inc, Bloomington, IN) is effective in active bleeding but is not available in the United States.

Endoscopic therapy is usually successful in postpolypectomy bleeding. If bleeding cannot be controlled at the time of endoscopy, salvage angiographic embolization should be considered as the next step. Endoscopically placed clips are effective markers of the bleeding site and facilitate subsequent supraselective angiographic embolization using microcoils to minimize the risk of colonic ischemia. Surgical intervention for torrential postpolypectomy hemorrhage is a rare occurrence.

Prevention of hemorrhage

Placement of a detachable snare (PolyLoop; Olympus Corp., Tokyo, Japan) or injection of epinephrine into the stalk of particularly large pedunculated polyps (≥2 cm) can significantly reduce bleeding AEs after snare polypectomy (Video 5).[20] Moreover, the combined use of epinephrine injection followed by detachable snare placement has been reported superior to epinephrine injection alone in decreasing the proportion of early postpolypectomy bleeding episodes in patients with large pedunculated polyps.[21] Placement of the detachable snare before polyp resection can be problematic for a pedunculated lesion with a large polyp head situated in a narrow lumen or at an angulated location. In addition, the detachable snare cannot be reopened once constrained and can become entangled inadvertently in the polyp head rather than the stalk, making subsequent attempts at snare resection difficult or impossible. For these reasons, prophylactic placement of the detachable snare following polyp transection is more desirable as long as a residual stalk of sufficient length is maintained. Detachable snares for large pedunculated polyps ($\geq$2 cm) with thick stalks should be considered in patients in need of antithrombotic therapy. Endoscopic clip placement across the base of the stalk is an alternative treatment option in the patient on antithrombotic therapy, provided that near complete cross-sectional compression of the stalk can be achieved. Contact between the clips and the snare results in transmission of the electrical coagulating current into the clip during polypectomy. In one randomized trial, prophylactic clip placement was as effective as the detachable snare in the prevention of postpolypectomy bleeding in large pedunculated polyps (Video 6).[22]

In two studies, prophylactic clip placement did not prevent delayed bleeding from postpolypectomy ulcers, although the mean size of the ulcers was small in one of the studies.[23,24] A retrospective study assessing the role of prophylactic clipping following resection of large flat or sessile polyps ($\geq$2 cm) suggested that not clipping the EMR defect was associated with an increased risk for delayed bleeding (OR, 6.0; 95% CI, 2.0–18.5).[15] Until more robust data are available to further define the role of prophylactic clip placement for large EMR defects, universal use of clips cannot be endorsed currently. However, consideration should be given for clipping EMR defects greater than 2 cm in size that either may have demonstrated oozing or contain an indeterminate focal (vascular) spot, particularly in the right colon and in patients who require immediate antithrombotic therapy to decrease the risk of postpolypectomy bleeding (**Fig. 3**).

Perforation

Iatrogenic colonic perforation is a serious AE. Perforation rates range from 0.01% to 0.8% for diagnostic colonoscopy, but can be 5% following therapeutic procedures, such as ESD.[25,26] Perforations occurring during resection (eg, EMR and ESD) tend to be smaller than perforating tears occurring during diagnostic colonoscopy and are more amenable to endoscopic closure. In one study, mean perforation diameters were 19.3 mm and 5.8 mm for diagnostic and therapeutic procedures, respectively.[27] In another study, laparotomy was required in 88% of perforations because of colonoscopic tears as opposed to only 9% of resection perforations.[28]

A key determinant for a successful outcome is immediate recognition and management of the perforation.[29] The perforation site can be inconspicuous, manifesting as a discreet mural defect without observable extraluminal fat, organs, or serosal tissue. Lack of recognition and continuation of the procedure with ongoing air insufflation may result in tension pneumoperitoneum, requiring percutaneous needle decompression to relieve discomfort and cardiorespiratory compromise.[30] Following dye-assisted EMR, the "target sign" signals a perforation with need for closure (**Fig. 4**).[31]

In the postprocedural setting, perforation should be considered and an appropriate work-up initiated in the presence of persistent abdominal pain. The absence of free air on plain films of the abdomen does not rule out perforation, and an abdominal computed tomography (CT) should be obtained when a high index of suspicion for perforation exists because CT is sensitive at detecting small-volume extraluminal or retroperitoneal air.

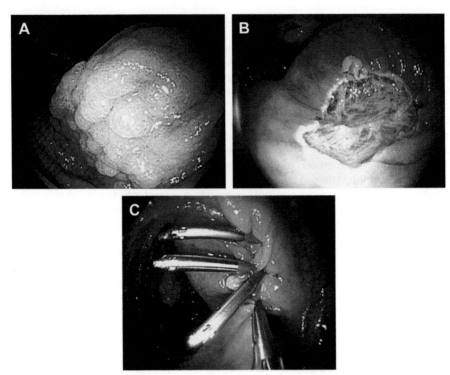

Fig. 3. (*A*) Large right-sided laterally spreading tumor of the granular type. (*B*) Postresection defect. (*C*) Prophylactic clip closure to prevent delayed bleeding.

Endoscopic closure versus operative repair

The decision to intervene operatively or to manage the perforation conservatively with endoscopic closure is influenced by the size and location of injury, quality of the bowel preparation, evidence for containment or extraluminal spillage, remaining pathology (ie, incomplete EMR), clinical stability of the patient, available devices, failure to access and completely close the perforation, and expertise (**Fig. 5**). Surgery is indicated in the presence of a large perforation, failed endoscopic closure, gross feculent peritoneal contamination, residual lesion, and clinical deterioration on conservative management. Perforations less than 1 to 2 cm in size are generally amenable to endoscopic closure in the setting of a relatively clean colon and controlled access to the perforated site. The patient should be positioned so that the perforation is opposite pooling of colonic contents. If available, CO_2 should be used for insufflation.

The decision to intervene surgically should be made within 24 hours after endoscopic closure if there is lack of significant improvement or the patient clinically deteriorates within that time frame because additional time delay affects surgical outcomes. Patients are more likely to receive a colostomy rather than primary repair or resection with anastomosis when the presentation is delayed (>24 hours).[32] A challenging situation is the delayed perforation, discovered by subsequent CT imaging performed for postprocedural pain in the recovery unit or beyond 24 hours. In many instances of delayed recognition of perforation during postprocedure recovery, these are microperforations and conservative management alone may suffice because these lesions can heal spontaneously by contraction of the colonic wall and sealing by pericolic tissue.[27] It remains undetermined if prompt repeat colonoscopy for

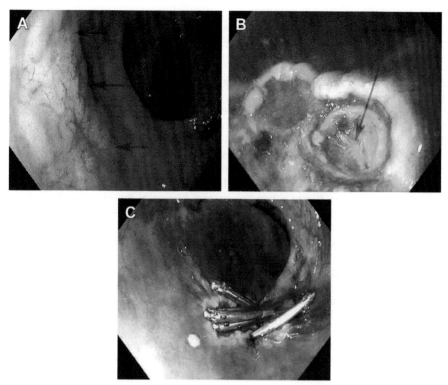

Fig. 4. (*A*) Large sessile polyp (*arrow*). (*B*) Target sign (*arrow*) apparent following piecemeal EMR. (*C*) Clip closure of target sign defect.

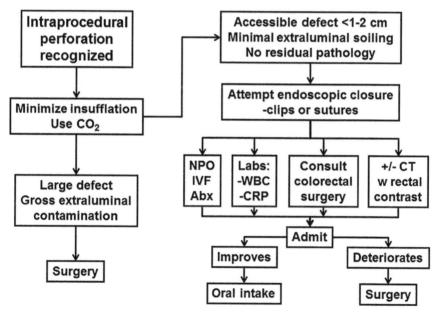

Fig. 5. Proposed management algorithm for an intraprocedurally recognized colonic perforation. Abx, antibiotics; CO_2, carbon dioxide; CRP, C-reactive protein; CT, computed tomography; IVF, intravenous fluids; NPO, nil per os; WBC, white blood count.

closure of radiologically proven microperforations results in better outcomes. Perforations diagnosed after 24 hours, especially those with CT findings of fluid collection, all require surgical intervention.

Endoscopic techniques for perforation closure

Through-the-scope mucosal clips are the most commonly used devices for closure of EMR and ESD perforations (**Fig. 6**). In the absence of a comparative study, the selection of a particular clip is based primarily on operator preference and device availability. Mucosal clips are generally successful at closing linear perforations less than or equal to 2 cm in size (**Fig. 7**, Video 7), although effective closure of larger, nongaping perforations has been reported.[33] Successful clip application is aided by the following: gentle suction, including the use of a cap, to approximate the margins of the perforation and capture more tissue within the opened blades of the clip; initiation of clip closure from left-to-right for a transverse perforation and top-to-bottom for a longitudinal perforation; and closely placing the clips to each other to ensure adequate closure and avoid leak from unsealed "dog ears" at either end of the perforation. The reported long-term success rates following mucosal clip closure of colonoscopic perforations from all causes range from 59% to 93%.[33–35]

Although mucosal clips can provide satisfactory closure of small perforations, they might not be adequate for larger defects with gaping holes because of their limited wingspan, low compression force, and potential for early detachment. In these situations, the OTSC might be more appropriate because of its ability to grasp more tissue and apply a greater compressive force with the potential for single layer full-thickness closure (**Fig. 8**). Moreover, grasping devices, such as the twin grasper and retractable nitinol tissue hooks, assist in capturing the defect margins and enable pulling them into the OTSC cap more reliably before clip deployment. Caution must be exercised to avoid inadvertent suction of adjacent organ into the OTSC cap. Drawing mesenteric fat into the cap along with the defect margins enhances effective closure (omental plug). The OTSC is successful at closing perforations that are less than 1 to 2 cm in size with noninflamed, nonfibrotic surrounding tissue, and treated within 24 hours.[36]

Through-the-Scope (TTS) Clips

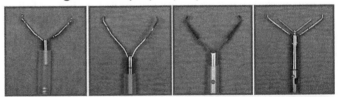

	QuickClip2	QuickClipPro	Resolution	Instinct
Jaw span	7 or 11 mm	11 mm	11 mm	16 mm
Rotation	Yes	Yes	No	Yes
Re-opening capability	No	Yes	Yes	Yes
Retention time (median)	2 wk	NA	4 wk	NA

Fig. 6. Endoscopic through-the-scope mucosal clips.

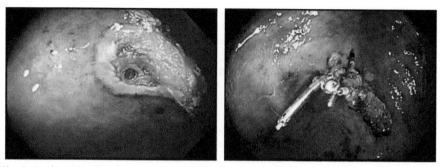

Fig. 7. Endoscopic clip closure of a small perforation following cecal polypectomy.

However, limitations of the OTSC device include the need to withdraw the endoscope to load the device (similar to a band ligator), the potential for mucosal lacerations and inability to maneuver the device through narrowed and angulated lumen (eg, sigmoid colon), and failure to reidentify the perforation site. The latter can be avoided by placing a tattoo or mucosal clip on the opposite wall of the perforation before scope withdrawal. The overall pooled estimates of procedural and clinical success were 89% and 80%, respectively, in a recent systematic review of various types of GI perforations closed with OTSC.[37]

Endoscopic suturing of perforations is an appealing concept for perforation closure. One endoscopic suturing device (OverStitch; Apollo Endosurgery, Austin, TX) is

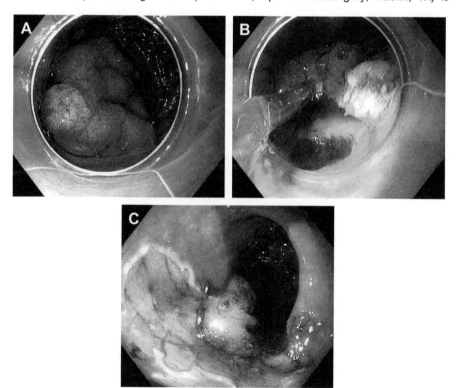

Fig. 8. (*A*) Large sessile rectal polyp. (*B*) Perforation during piecemeal EMR. (*C*) Over-the-scope clip closure of perforation following completion EMR.

currently available on the market, but requires a double-channel upper endoscope (GIF 2T160 or GIF2TH-180; Olympus Corp., Tokyo, Japan) for its use. The device is capable of deploying multiple interrupted or running stitches for accurate full-thickness closure, and has been used to prophylactically close very large rectal EMR and ESD defects deemed not amenable to standard clip closure for prevention of delayed perforation and bleeding (Video 8).[38] It is used for closure of full-thickness resection sites and perforations. Related limitations include the need for a specialized double-channel upper endoscope, inability to treat lesions beyond the reach of the endoscope, and restricted maneuverability caused by instrument design and colon anatomy. Other suturing devices have been described in the experimental setting and in small case series, but are not currently marketed for endoscopic closure.[39] The single-layer full-thickness closure with serosa-to-serosa apposition is superior to those that provide mucosa-to-mucosa apposition.[40]

Postprocedural monitoring and management

A multidisciplinary approach is essential in the postendoscopic closure care of the patient. Initial management consists of bowel rest; intravenous fluids; broad-spectrum antibiotics covering gut organisms; and clinical monitoring for tachycardia, fever, leukocytosis, and diffuse peritoneal signs on serial abdominal examination (see **Fig. 5**).

The endoscopic appearance of a secured closure is not predictive of long-term success because incomplete clip closure, clip loss, inaccurate stitch placement, and superficial stitch dehiscence can occur; hence, there is a need for close monitoring for clinical deterioration. Some institutions incorporate a CT with rectal administration of water-soluble contrast in their management algorithms for perforation to confirm absence of leak after endoscopic closure,[41] although there is a theoretic risk for increasing intraluminal colonic pressure and undoing the perforation repair with contrast instillation. In the situation where clinical progress is ambiguous, the decision to intervene surgically is a difficult one, and surgery might be delayed beyond the optimal period ($\leq$24 hours). An abdominal CT at this moment might be useful because such findings as extraluminal accumulation of fluid and debris suggest persistent leak and should elicit prompt surgical exploration.

Oral intake can resume as soon as pain and fever subside; bowel function returns; and laboratory indices of inflammation, such as leukocytosis and elevated C-reactive protein levels, normalize. Patients whose course remains uneventful typically are able to consume liquids at 48 hours after the procedure, with subsequent gradual advancement to a normal diet.

Postpolypectomy Syndrome

PPS is secondary to transmural thermal injury without perforation following snare resection. This AE occurs in up to 3% of patients undergoing hot snare polypectomy.[42] PPS occurs most often after resection of large (>2 cm) sessile polyps, particularly in the thin-walled right colon, with long duration application of electrosurgical current (coagulation mode primarily). In one study, hypertension, large lesion size, and nonpolypoid configuration of the lesion were independently associated with PPS.[42] The use of a submucosal fluid cushion during EMR may reduce, but does not eliminate, the risk of PPS.[43]

As a result of serosal irritation and localized peritonitis, patients can present within hours and up to 5 days postprocedure with localized abdominal pain and peritoneal signs, fever, and leukocytosis that mimic colonic perforation. Abdominal CT is the best radiologic test at distinguishing PPS from perforation, and the findings of localized colonic wall thickening and adjacent fat stranding without extraluminal air are consistent with PPS.

Management is supportive and consists of bowel rest, intravenous fluids, antibiotics, and pain control in those who require hospitalization. Patients with mild symptoms and adequate outpatient follow-up can be managed with oral antibiotics and a clear liquid diet for 1 to 2 days. The prognosis for PPS is excellent.

SUMMARY

AEs from EMR, ESD, and polypectomy include immediate and delayed bleeding, immediate and delayed perforation, and PPS. Risk factors for bleeding include large flat or sessile lesions, large pedunculated polyps with thick stalks, lesion location in the right colon, mode of electrosurgical current used, and anticoagulation status. Consideration should be given for prophylactic maneuvers, such as clip and detachable snare placement, to prevent bleeding when faced with these high-risk patients and lesions. Immediate bleeding can be managed effectively with a variety of therapies including clips and thermal coagulation, with or without epinephrine injection. Delayed bleeding can be managed conservatively in most cases, but may require endoscopic intervention in the presence of recurrent or ongoing bleeding. Immediate recognition and closure of polypectomy-, EMR-, or ESD-induced perforation are key determinants for a successful outcome. Standard through-the-scope mucosal clip placement constitutes the mainstay of endoscopic therapy for perforation, although OTSC and suturing may be more appropriate for select lesions. Close monitoring post perforation closure is essential in the context of a multidisciplinary approach, with prompt surgical intervention in the presence of clinical deterioration, fluid collections, and in the setting of delayed perforation beyond 24 hours. PPS is the result of transmural injury without perforation during snare electrocautery and has an excellent outcome with conservative management.

SUPPLEMENTARY DATA

Supplementary data related to this article can be found online at http://dx.doi.org/10.1016/j.giec.2014.09.007.

REFERENCES

1. Whitlock EP, Lin JS, Liles E, et al. Screening for colorectal cancer: a targeted, updated systematic review for the U.S. Preventive Services Task Force. Ann Intern Med 2008;149:638–58.
2. Morris ML, Tucker RD, Baron TH, et al. Electrosurgery in gastrointestinal endoscopy: principles to practice. Am J Gastroenterol 2009;104:1563–74.
3. Hsieh YH, Lin HJ, Tseng GY, et al. Is submucosal epinephrine injection necessary before polypectomy? A prospective, comparative study. Hepatogastroenterology 2001;48:1379–82.
4. Lee SH, Chung IK, Kim SJ, et al. Comparison of postpolypectomy bleeding between epinephrine and saline submucosal injection for large colon polyps by conventional polypectomy: a prospective randomized, multicenter study. World J Gastroenterol 2007;13:2973–7.
5. Moss A, Bourke MJ, Metz AJ. A randomized, double-blind trial of succinylated gelatin submucosal injection for endoscopic resection of large sessile polyps of the colon. Am J Gastroenterol 2010;105:2375–82.
6. ASGE Standards of Practice Committee, Fisher DA, Maple JT, et al. Complications of colonoscopy. Gastrointest Endosc 2011;74:745–52.

7. Day LW, Kwon A, Inadomi JM, et al. Adverse events in older patients undergoing colonoscopy: a systematic review and meta-analysis. Gastrointest Endosc 2011; 74:885–96.
8. Rabeneck L, Saskin R, Paszat LF. Onset and clinical course of bleeding and perforation after outpatient colonoscopy: a population-based study. Gastrointest Endosc 2011;73:520–3.
9. Ko CW, Dominitz JA. Complications of colonoscopy: magnitude and management. Gastrointest Endosc Clin N Am 2010;20:659–71.
10. Watabe H, Yamaji Y, Okamoto M, et al. Risk assessment for delayed hemorrhagic complication of colonic polypectomy: polyp-related factors and patient-related factors. Gastrointest Endosc 2006;64:73–8.
11. Conio M, Ponchon T, Blanchi S, et al. Endoscopic mucosal resection. Am J Gastroenterol 2006;101:653–63.
12. Burgess NG, Metz AJ, Williams SJ, et al. Risk factors for intraprocedural and clinically significant delayed bleeding after wide-field endoscopic mucosal resection of large colonic lesions. Clin Gastroenterol Hepatol 2014;12:651–61.
13. Kim HS, Kim TI, Kim WH, et al. Risk factors for immediate postpolypectomy bleeding of the colon: a multicenter study. Am J Gastroenterol 2006;101:1333–41.
14. Buddingh KT, Herngreen T, Haringsma J, et al. Location in the right hemi-colon is an independent risk factor for delayed post-polypectomy hemorrhage: a multicenter case-control study. Am J Gastroenterol 2011;106:1119–24.
15. Liaquat H, Rohn E, Rex DK. Prophylactic clip closure reduced the risk of delayed postpolypectomy hemorrhage: experience in 277 clipped large sessile or flat colorectal lesions and 247 control lesions. Gastrointest Endosc 2013;77:401–7.
16. Hui AJ, Wong RM, Ching JY, et al. Risk of colonoscopic polypectomy bleeding with anticoagulants and antiplatelet agents: analysis of 1657 cases. Gastrointest Endosc 2004;59:44–8.
17. Gandhi S, Narula N, Mosleh W, et al. Meta-analysis: colonoscopic postpolypectomy bleeding in patients on continued clopidogrel therapy. Aliment Pharmacol Ther 2013;37:947–52.
18. Feagins LA, Uddin FS, Davila RE, et al. The rate of post-polypectomy bleeding for patients on uninterrupted clopidogrel therapy during elective colonoscopy is acceptably low. Dig Dis Sci 2011;56:2631–8.
19. Van Gossum A, Cozzoli A, Adler M, et al. Colonoscopic snare polypectomy: analysis of 1485 resections comparing two types of current. Gastrointest Endosc 1992;38:472–5.
20. Di Giorgio P, De Luca L, Calcagno G, et al. Detachable snare versus epinephrine injection in the prevention of postpolypectomy bleeding: a randomized and controlled study. Endoscopy 2004;36:860–3.
21. Paspatis GA, Paraskeva K, Theodoropoulou A, et al. A prospective, randomized comparison of adrenaline injection in combination with detachable snare versus adrenaline injection alone in the prevention of postpolypectomy bleeding in large colonic polyps. Am J Gastroenterol 2006;101:2805 [quiz: 2913].
22. Ji JS, Lee SW, Kim TH, et al. Comparison of prophylactic clip and endoloop application for the prevention of postpolypectomy bleeding in pedunculated colonic polyps: a prospective, randomized, multicenter study. Endoscopy 2014;46:598–604.
23. Shioji K, Suzuki Y, Kobayashi M, et al. Prophylactic clip application does not decrease delayed bleeding after colonoscopic polypectomy. Gastrointest Endosc 2003;57:691–4.
24. Feagins LA, Nguyen AD, Iqbal R, et al. The prophylactic placement of hemoclips to prevent delayed post-polypectomy bleeding: an unnecessary practice? A case control study. Dig Dis Sci 2014;59(4):823–8.

25. Panteris V, Haringsma J, Kuipers EJ. Colonoscopy perforation rate, mechanisms and outcome: from diagnostic to therapeutic colonoscopy. Endoscopy 2009;41:941–51.
26. Lohsiriwat V. Colonoscopic perforation: incidence, risk factors, management and outcome. World J Gastroenterol 2010;16:425–30.
27. Yang DH, Byeon JS, Lee KH, et al. Is endoscopic closure with clips effective for both diagnostic and therapeutic colonoscopy-associated bowel perforation? Surg Endosc 2010;24:1177–85.
28. Avgerinos DV, Llaguna OH, Lo AY, et al. Evolving management of colonoscopic perforations. J Gastrointest Surg 2008;12:1783–9.
29. Raju GS, Saito Y, Matsuda T, et al. Endoscopic management of colonoscopic perforations (with videos). Gastrointest Endosc 2011;74:1380–8.
30. Baron TH, Wong Kee Song LM, Zielinski MD, et al. A comprehensive approach to the management of acute endoscopic perforations (with videos). Gastrointest Endosc 2012;76:838–59.
31. Swan MP, Bourke MJ, Moss A, et al. The target sign: an endoscopic marker for the resection of the muscularis propria and potential perforation during colonic endoscopic mucosal resection. Gastrointest Endosc 2010;73:79–85.
32. Iqbal CW, Cullinane DC, Schiller HJ, et al. Surgical management and outcomes of 165 colonoscopic perforations from a single institution. Arch Surg 2008;143:701–7.
33. Trecca A, Gaj F, Gagliardi G. Our experience with endoscopic repair of large colonoscopic perforations and review of the literature. Tech Coloproctol 2008;12:315–21.
34. Cho SB, Lee WS, Joo YE, et al. Therapeutic options for iatrogenic colon perforation: feasibility of endoscopic clip closure and predictors of the need for early surgery. Surg Endosc 2012;26:473–9.
35. Kim JS, Kim BW, Kim JI, et al. Endoscopic clip closure versus surgery for the treatment of iatrogenic colon perforations developed during diagnostic colonoscopy: a review of 115,285 patients. Surg Endosc 2013;27:501–4.
36. Hagel AF, Naegel A, Lindner AS, et al. Over-the-scope clip application yields a high rate of closure in gastrointestinal perforations and may reduce emergency surgery. J Gastrointest Surg 2012;16:2132–8.
37. Weiland T, Fehlker M, Gottwald T, et al. Performance of the OTSC system in the endoscopic closure of iatrogenic gastrointestinal perforations: a systematic review. Surg Endosc 2013;27:2258–74.
38. Kantsevoy SV, Bitner M, Mitrakov AA, et al. Endoscopic suturing closure of large mucosal defects after endoscopic submucosal dissection and eliminates the need for hospitalization (with videos). Gastrointest Endosc 2014;79:503–7.
39. Banerjee S, Barth BA, Bhat YM, et al. Endoscopic closure devices. Gastrointest Endosc 2012;76:244–51.
40. Voermans RP, Le Moine O, von Renteln D, et al. Efficacy of endoscopic closure of acute perforations of the gastrointestinal tract. Clin Gastroenterol Hepatol 2012;10:603–8.
41. Kowalczyk L, Forsmark CE, Ben-David K, et al. Algorithm for the management of endoscopic perforations: a quality improvement project. Am J Gastroenterol 2011;106:1022–7.
42. Cha JM, Lim KS, Lee SH, et al. Clinical outcomes and risk factors of post-polypectomy coagulation syndrome: a multicenter, retrospective, case-control study. Endoscopy 2013;45:202–7.
43. Ferrara F, Luigiano C, Ghersi S, et al. Efficacy, safety and outcomes of "inject and cut" endoscopic mucosal resection for large sessile and flat colorectal polyps. Digestion 2010;82:213–20.

Adverse Events Associated with Percutaneous Enteral Access

Ajaypal Singh, MD, Andres Gelrud, MD, MMSc*

KEYWORDS

- Percutaneous endoscopic gastrostomy
- Direct percutaneous endoscopic jejunostomy • Adverse events
- Endoscopic enteral access

KEY POINTS

- There is a high incidence of complications after percutaneous enteral access but most are minor.
- There is a high mortality in patients undergoing percutaneous enteral access but this is usually caused by underlying illness.
- American Society for Gastrointestinal Endoscopy guidelines exist regarding the use of antibiotics and management of antithrombotics and anticoagulation before percutaneous endoscopic gastrostomies but data about other complications are limited.
- Careful patient selection is imperative and should involve detailed evaluation of indications, contraindications, risks and benefits, possible technical difficulties, and ethical issues involved with long-term enteral access.

MINIMIZING THE ADVERSE EVENTS ASSOCIATED WITH PERCUTANEOUS ENTERAL ACCESS

Percutaneous endoscopic enteral access is required in patients who need long-term enteral nutrition or decompression of the gastrointestinal tract for distal obstruction. It can be achieved by various modalities and includes the most commonly used percutaneous endoscopic gastrostomy (PEG) along with placement of direct jejunostomy (DPEJ) or placement of a jejunal extension through the PEG (PEG-J). The technique of PEG placement without the need for a laparotomy was first described in 1980 by Gauderer and Ponsky.[1,2] Since then there have been numerous modifications and although the procedure-related mortality is low (less than 1%),[3] several studies

Disclosures: None.
Division of Gastroenterology, Center for Endoscopic Research and Therapeutics (CERT), University of Chicago Medical Center, 5700 Sought Maryland Ave, Chicago, IL 60637-1470, USA
* Corresponding author.
E-mail address: agelrud@bsd.uchicago.edu

Gastrointest Endoscopy Clin N Am 25 (2015) 71–82
http://dx.doi.org/10.1016/j.giec.2014.09.003
1052-5157/15/$ – see front matter © 2015 Elsevier Inc. All rights reserved.

have reported short-term mortality in these patients ranging from 10% to 25%.[4,5] A recent study showed decreased 30-day and 1-year mortality rates in patients who received PEG compared with those who were offered but deferred PEG placement.[6] In a recent multicenter study from South Korea involving 1625 patients undergoing PEG placement with pull technique, the overall complication rate was reported to be 13% with most of these being minor.[3] Earlier studies done in the United States have shown complication rates ranging from 13% to 32%.[7–9] Even though the procedure-related mortality and morbidity are low, overall mortality is high in these patients (approaching 24% at 1-year in one study) and is usually related to underlying medical conditions.[5] These findings were confirmed by a recent study from Europe in which it was shown that 24-week mortality in patients undergoing PEG placement depended on the indication and was significantly higher in patients who underwent PEG placement for neurologic reasons compared with those with tumor-related indications (60% vs 27.7%, respectively).[10]

ADVERSE EVENTS ASSOCIATED WITH UPPER ENDOSCOPY

Most of the data about complications related to upper endoscopy are obtained from relatively healthy patients who undergo the procedure in an outpatient setting, whereas PEG placement is commonly performed in relatively sicker patients with much higher comorbidities and lower life expectancy. The adverse events associated with upper endoscopy and their management strategies are discussed elsewhere in this issue and are not discussed here.

PNEUMOPERITONEUM AND PERITONITIS

Pneumoperitoneum is reportedly common after PEG placement and is usually a temporary and benign condition. Previous studies have shown an incidence of around 40% for endoscopic and around 55% for radiologically placed gastrostomies.[11,12] In a prospective study involving 65 patients undergoing PEG placement, pneumoperitoneum was noted on radiographs in 20% of patients at 3 hours. Most of these resolved but pneumoperitoneum persisted in three patients beyond 72 hours without any clinical significance in any of these patients.[13] In a retrospective study, Blum and colleagues[14] showed that free intra-abdominal air was noted in 12% of patients on radiographic imaging within 5 days of PEG or PEG-J placement. A total of 85% of these patients did not have any complications, whereas 15% developed signs and symptoms concerning for peritonitis and required laparotomy. Hence clinical condition postprocedure should dictate management rather than the finding of free air that is of no clinical significance in most cases.

In a retrospective review of 322 surgical intensive care unit patients undergoing PEG placement, 5% developed peritonitis requiring laparotomy.[15] Body mass index higher than 30 kg/m^2 and serum albumin lower than 2.5 gm/dL were associated with increased risk of peritonitis. Use of carbon dioxide for insufflation during PEG placement has been shown to be associated with lower incidence of pneumoperitoneum and lesser distention of small bowel.[16]

ASPIRATION

Aspiration is one of the most common major complications related to the placement of PEG tubes and can occur during or after the procedure. The rate of aspiration events occurring periprocedurally has been reported to be around 1%, whereas postprocedure aspiration has been reported in up to 20% to 30% of patients and is associated with high mortality.[7,17] Most of the periprocedural aspiration events are related to aspiration of oropharyngeal contents, whereas delayed aspiration events also involve gastric contents including tube feeds. Periprocedural aspiration events can be affected by the depth of sedation, frequency of suctioning during procedure, and level of head elevation. All of these should be closely monitored and optimized during all endoscopic procedures. Postprocedural aspiration events have been shown to be related to the presence of reflux esophagitis, hiatal hernia, and impaired swallowing, the last one being an indication itself for PEG placement in many of these patients.[18] Placement of PEG tubes for prevention of aspiration pneumonia in patients with cognitive impairment is not supported by present literature because there are no conclusive data that PEG feedings decrease aspiration rates.[19,20]

INJURY TO ADJACENT VISCERA

Because placement of a PEG tube relies on transillumination and finding the site of insertion by finger indentation on the abdominal wall, there is a very low risk of injury to the organs adjacent to the anterior abdominal wall including colon,[21,22] small bowel, liver, and spleen.[23–25] These adverse events are uncommon and hence exact incidence is not known but there are multiple case reports. Bowel injury in patients undergoing PEG placement is usually seen in very young or elderly patients because of laxity of the mesentery that can lead to bowel transposition between the abdominal wall and anterior wall of the stomach. Excessive insufflation of the stomach and small bowel can also lead to gastric rotation and bowel transposition. Making sure that there is 1:1 indentation before needle insertion can prevent this event. The needle should always be advanced into the gastric lumen under direct endoscopic visualization while pulling back on the syringe as the needle is advanced. Free suction of air is noted at the same time as the needle is visualized in the stomach; this ensures the air being suctioned is not coming from the bowel lumen.

Although some published reports indicate that transhepatic insertion can be managed conservatively, there is a case report describing massive intraperitoneal bleeding caused by liver injury.[23] Colonic injury during PEG insertion can be initially asymptomatic and difficult to diagnose clinically unless there is a high clinical suspicion but can lead to formation of cologastric or colocutaneous fistulas over time (described later).

BLEEDING

Placement of endoscopic gastrostomy or jejunostomy tubes can lead to early bleeding from the abdominal wall or delayed bleeding from ulcer formation. In a retrospective review of 1625 patients with PEG placement in South Korea, 1.2% of patients developed bleeding.[3] Use of anticoagulant agents and the presence of diabetes mellitus were associated with an increased risk of bleeding. Two retrospective reviews involving more than 1000 patients each from the United States showed post–PEG placement bleeding rates ranging from 2.8% to 3.3%.[26,27] Immediate gastric bleeding after PEG placement is usually caused by an injury to the gastroepiploic artery itself or one of its branches. It can be controlled by external pressure at the PEG site. Sometimes tightening of the PEG bumper against the abdominal wall is needed to tamponade the bleeding. However, it is important to loosen the bumper after 48 hours to prevent ischemic injury and ulceration of the gastric mucosa at the PEG site. Severe intraperitoneal hemorrhage can occur because of liver laceration and presents as severe postprocedure hypotension with or without peritonitis. The management is primarily surgical and it has high mortality based on the scant data from case reports.[23,28]

American Society for Gastrointestinal Endoscopy Standards of Practice Committee 2009 guidelines consider PEG placement a high-risk procedure for gastrointestinal bleeding and hence recommend holding newer antiplatelet medications (theinopyridines) for 7 to 10 days before the procedure in patients who are low risk for cardiovascular complications. In patients who are high risk for cardiovascular complications, PEG placement should be deferred until it is safe to hold anticoagulation and antiplatelet therapy and alternate methods for feeding should be considered.[29] Those patients who are on anticoagulation should have their anticoagulation held and bridging with short-acting anticoagulants should be considered. Nonsteroidal anti-inflammatory drugs and aspirin can be continued before PEG placement.

Common endoscopic findings in patients undergoing endoscopy for upper gastrointestinal bleeding after PEG placement include reflux esophagitis (most common finding in two studies), mucosal tears, and gastric erosions or ulcers.[20,30] Gastric ulceration from PEG placement can occur on anterior and posterior walls of the stomach. Anterior ulceration is usually caused by pressure necrosis from excessive tension between the bumper and face plate. It is of great importance to evaluate the mucosa below the gastric bumper or balloon after external manipulation during the endoscopy (**Fig. 1**). Excessive traction should be avoided to prevent these ulcers after PEG placement and it is our practice to loosen the bumper by 1 cm approximately 24 hours after PEG placement to ensure it is freely rotating at the skin surface.

INFECTIONS

Infectious complications are common without the routine use of prophylactic antibiotics, with one study reporting an incidence of around 38%.[31] Most of the infections are minor and include local wound infections but serious infections including peritonitis and necrotizing fasciitis can also occur after PEG placement. In a randomized clinical trial, Ahmad and colleagues[32] showed that use of periprocedural antibiotics decreased the risk of peristomal infections in the first week after PEG placement

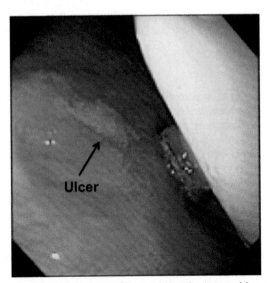

Fig. 1. Endoscopic view of an ulcer (*arrow*) seen under the internal bumper of a PEG tube. The patient presented with melena multiple months after PEG placement.

from 18% to 3%. A meta-analysis of 10 randomized controlled trials involving more than 1000 patients showed that penicillin- and cephalosporin-based prophylaxis are effective in decreasing the risk of wound infections after PEG placement.[33] Overall relative risk reduction was 64% with absolute risk reduction of 15% and number needed to treat was 8 to prevent one wound infection. Penicillin-based prophylaxis was slightly superior to cephalosporin-based prophylaxis (absolute risk reduction of 13% vs 10% and number needed to treat 8 vs 10). Current American Society for Gastrointestinal Endoscopy guidelines recommend parental cefazolin (or an antibiotic with equivalent coverage) to be administered in all patients 30 minutes before PEG placement.[34] With the increasing prevalence of methicillin-resistant *Staphylococcus aureus* (MRSA) colonization in hospitalized patients, MRSA wound infections have been recognized as an important cause of gastrostomy wound infections. Thomas and colleagues[35] have shown that MRSA screening before PEG placement and subsequent decontamination can decrease the incidence of MRSA wound infections but more conclusive data are needed before this can be recommended in all patients undergoing PEG placement. An important factor to prevent the local infectious complications is adherence to sterile technique.

Most of the gastrostomy wound infections can be managed by local wound care but close monitoring to make sure that it does not progress to deep tissue involvement is important. Necrotizing fasciitis is a rare but potentially fatal complication that can occur from infection at the PEG site. Most of the cases of necrotizing fasciitis have been documented as case reports[36–40] and hence actual incidence is not known. Management of necrotizing fasciitis involves surgical debridement along with broad antibiotic coverage and is associated with high morbidity and mortality.

BURIED BUMPER SYNDROME

Buried bumper refers to displacement of the gastrostomy tube internal bumper into the PEG tract anywhere between the gastric and anterior abdominal walls. It is a rare but serious complication with reported incidence of 0.3% to 2.4% in most studies,[41,42] although one study reported an incidence of 9%.[43] Buried bumpers usually present with leakage of tube feeds around the PEG site, inability to push feeds through the PEG, pain and swelling at the site, and in some cases with frank peritonitis (**Fig. 2**). The diagnosis should be highly suspected in patients who have pain out of proportion to the abdominal examination findings and in those with signs of peritonitis and can be confirmed by either endoscopy or by computed tomography scan that can show the exact location of the bumper. All buried bumpers should be removed, even in asymptomatic patients. Sometimes the PEG can be removed by using the pull technique only or it can be pushed back in to the stomach (if the location is intramural) but in cases of subcutaneous infections or extramural location of the bumper, surgical intervention is needed. There are some case reports that have shown removal of buried bumper by inserting a through-the-scope balloon dilator and inflating it over a wire before pulling the tube out of the patient's mouth[44] or by making a small gastric incision using a needle knife.[43,45] The main reason for the buried bumper is believed to be excessive traction between the bumper and the abdominal wall face plate leading to pressure necrosis and subsequent migration. The factors that can contribute to this process include tightening of the bumper after placement, weight gain after PEG placement, obesity, chronic cough (leading to increased intra-abdominal pressure), and placement of gauze or bandage below the external skin bumper to keep the site clean and dry adding tension to the bumper. We recommend that the external skin

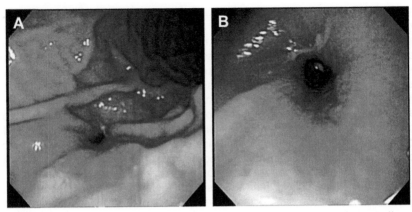

Fig. 2. Buried bumper syndrome. (*A*) The internal bumper is not visible endoscopically and a mucosal defect is noted. (*B*) Closer view of the site of buried bumper. Only a part of the bumper was visible inside the defect. The PEG tube was successfully removed endoscopically.

bumper should always be kept loose and easily rotatable at the skin site to prevent buried bumper and ischemic ulceration.

FISTULA FORMATION

If a PEG tube is inadvertently placed through the colon, there will be formation of a tract between the gastric wall and colon and between the colon and skin. This can be asymptomatic clinically but when the tube is removed or replaced with a percutaneously inserted gastrostomy tube, the gastrocolonic fistula is evident and the new tube also ends in the transverse colon. This can manifest as diarrhea after starting tube feeds through the replacement tube. The colocutaneous fistula is usually diagnosed radiographically by injecting dye through the new tube but can also be diagnosed endoscopically. Because PEG tubes are usually replaced after formation of fibrous tract, there is usually no spillage of contents into the peritoneum and hence no peritonitis. Initial studies showed an incidence of 2% to 3% for this complication but recent data suggest that the incidence is likely less than 1%.[46] These fistula tracts heal without consequences in most cases after removal of the tube. If the need for tube feeds persists, another PEG tube should be placed. Special care should be taken to avoid colonic injury during PEG placement by avoiding extra insufflation of stomach and small bowel. Because many patients requiring PEG placement have structural deformities of the spine and chronic constipation, both of which predispose the transverse colon to move in front of the anterior gastric wall, we obtain abdominal radiographs preprocedurally in most patients and give enemas to decompress the colon in patients with severe constipation and/or transverse colon overlying the stomach on radiographs.

GASTRIC OUTLET OBSTRUCTION

Gastric outlet obstruction is an infrequent adverse event after PEG placement and is mainly seen in pediatric patients when the internal bumper migrates distally and causes obstruction of the pyloric channel. It usually happens in adults after replacement of a bumper-type gastrostomy tube by a tube with an internal balloon with migration of the balloon into the pylorus or proximal small bowel.[47–50] These patients usually present with abdominal discomfort and nausea or vomiting and the gastric outlet obstruction can be diagnosed radiographically. It is avoided by proper positioning of the bumper to minimize the length of tube inside the gastric lumen while avoiding too much tension at the PEG site. Gastroduodenal intussusception caused by the internal bumper of gastrostomy tubes acting as lead point has been known to occur in children but no such cases have been reported in adults.[51,52]

TUMOR SEEDING

Enteral feeding tubes are commonly placed in patients with dysphagia caused by head, neck, and esophageal cancers. Seeding of the gastrostomy tract with tumor cells and subsequent development of tumor at the stoma site is a dreaded complication with reported incidence of 0.5% to 1%.[53–55] Exfoliated cells from these predominantly squamous cell cancers implant more readily at the PEG exit site (abdominal wall with squamous epithelium) than at the gastric site (columnar mucosa). Skin metastases indicates a poor prognosis with reported 1-year survival of 0% in the otolaryngology literature.[56] Cappell[53] reviewed all reported 44 cases of gastrostomy metastases after PEG placement and found that the metastases were detected after a mean period of 7.8 months (range, 3–30 months) after PEG insertion. Risk factors associated with tumor seeding included squamous cell histology, advanced cancer stage, poorly differentiated histology, untreated primary cancer, and use of pull technique compared with push technique. Even though direct implantation of tumor cells from manipulation during the procedure is the most commonly accepted explanation for this seeding phenomenon, hematogenous tumor spread has also been proposed as an alternative explanation.[54,55] Currently there are no guidelines to address this issue and help select patients with low risk of tumor seeding. It is important to discuss the low but real risk of tumor implantation in all patients with pharyngoesophageal malignancy undergoing PEG placement along with discussion of other options including using an overtube, placement of feeding tube using the push tube by radiology,[57] or delaying gastrostomy placement until surgical resection or chemotherapy, although there are no data to support any of these practices.

TUBE DISLODGEMENT

The reported 7-day dislodgment incidence after PEG placement is 4.1% and the lifetime incidence of this adverse event is 7.8%[58] with rates up to 20% in the pediatric population.[59] It is a frequent cause of health care visits, especially in patients with altered mental status or cognitive impairment and each replacement can cost an average of $1200.[58]

In most cases, the tract between the gastric and abdominal walls matures in a couple of weeks after PEG placement but it can take up to 4 weeks in patients who are malnourished or have other risk factors that can predispose to poor healing. If PEG tube dislodgement occurs after 4 weeks of initial placement, a replacement PEG tube can be placed through the same tract without the need for endoscopy. If a new PEG tube is not available immediately, a Foley or a red rubber catheter can be placed temporarily to keep the tract patent. In case of dislodgement within the first 4 weeks of placement, it should be assumed that the tract between stomach and abdominal walls has not matured and a repeat endoscopy is warranted for placement of a new tube either through the previously existing tract or via a new site. Removal of a PEG tube before the tract is mature also can lead to leakage of gastric contents into the peritoneum and patients should be closely watched for any signs of peritonitis.[58]

If a gastrostomy tube is not replaced immediately in these patients, they should be managed by keeping them nothing-by-mouth status, with nasogastric tube placement with suctioning of gastric contents and initiation of broad-spectrum antibiotics while working toward tube replacement as early as possible. Surgical intervention is needed if peritonitis develops. Blindly placing a new PEG in the absence of a mature tract can lead to the internal bumper ending up in the peritoneum and hence causing peritonitis.

Some factors that should be considered to decrease tube dislodgement and its associated complications include use of T-fasteners, limiting the length of the external portion of the gastrostomy tube, and use of low profile "button" gastrostomy tubes. However, there are no conclusive data to support the use of these strategies.

ADDITIONAL CONSIDERATIONS FOR DIRECT PERCUTANEOUS ENDOSCOPIC JEJUNOSTOMY AND PERCUTANEOUS ENDOSCOPIC GASTROSTOMY WITH JEJUNAL EXTENSION

Although most of the published literature suggests no decrease in aspiration rates in patients receiving gastric feedings, some studies have shown that postpyloric feeding does decrease this incidence. Furthermore, postpyloric or postligament of Treitz feeding is desired in certain conditions, such as gastric obstruction, gastroparesis, or pancreatitis. This can be achieved by either placing a PEG-J or by placing a DPEJ. Both of these techniques have their own issues and potential adverse events in addition to those mentioned previously for endoscopic gastrostomy. A few studies have shown decreased aspiration rates and decreased occlusion rates requiring reintervention in patients with DPEJs compared with those with PEG-Js.[60,61] PEG-J tubes are associated with complications that include occlusion (smaller lumen of the jejunal extension tube) and proximal dislodgement of the jejunal extension into the duodenum or stomach. Fan and colleagues[61] showed that approximately 56% of patients with PEG-J placement required repeat endoscopy within 6 months of placement to maintain jejunal access. Proximal migration of the jejunal extender was the cause in around 40% of these patients followed by tube occlusion (16%), tube leakage (16%), dislodged PEG (10%) bumper, inadvertent removal (5%), infection (5%), and unspecified tube dysfunction (5%).

Patients who had a DPEJ placement had a much lower rate of repeat endoscopy (13.5%) and much longer tube patency, but DPEJ placement was successful in only 72% of patients, whereas PEG-J was successfully placed in 92.5% of patients. Some authors have also proposed clipping the distal end to prevent proximal migration. DPEJ is technically difficult to place because of failure to transilluminate in many of the patients but scope looping and small bowel peristalsis can also contribute to this difficulty. PEG-J patency rates are improved by using a bigger jejunal extender tube especially if there is no need for gastric suctioning or decompression. In a retrospective review of 286 DPEJ placements, success was achieved in 68% of patients with adverse events occurring in 22.5% of cases. Although most of these adverse events were mild (site infection and persistent pain), moderate or serious adverse events were noted in 10% of patients and included bowel perforation (2.5%), serious bleeding, jejunal volvulus, chronic enterocutaneous fistulae, and aspiration.[62] One patient died because of intraperitoneal hemorrhage complicated by abdominal compartment syndrome after DPEJ placement. Using fluoroscopy to confirm that the endoscope is past the ligament of Treitz can facilitate placement of DPEJ.

SUMMARY

Although the placement of PEG or jejunostomy is a safe procedure with low peri-procedural mortality, overall mortality rates are high because of underlying disease conditions. These procedures are also associated with postprocedure complications, most of which are minor and can be easily managed. The clinically significant adverse events related to the procedures include infection (at tube site and peritonitis), bleeding, and aspiration. More rare associated events include buried bumpers, injury to adjacent viscera with subsequent fistula formation, and tumor seeding. It is important for the endoscopist to be aware of the potential for these adverse events to better recognize and treat them. There is still a lack of guidelines about these procedures other than those concerning the use of antibiotics and the management of antithrombotics and anticoagulation before the procedure.

REFERENCES

1. Ponsky JL, Gauderer MW. Percutaneous endoscopic gastrostomy: a non-operative technique for feeding gastrostomy. Gastrointest Endosc 1981;27: 9–11.
2. Gauderer MW, Ponsky JL, Izant RJ Jr. Gastrostomy without laparotomy: a percutaneous endoscopic technique. J Pediatr Surg 1980;15:872–5.
3. Small Intestine Research Group of the Korean Association for the Study of Intestinal Disease (KASID), Lee C, Im JP, et al. Risk factors for complications and mortality of percutaneous endoscopic gastrostomy: a multicenter, retrospective study. Surg Endosc 2013;27:3806–15.
4. Arora G, Rockey D, Gupta S. High in-hospital mortality after percutaneous endoscopic gastrostomy: results of a nationwide population-based study. Clin Gastroenterol Hepatol 2013;11:1437–44.e3.
5. Grant MD, Rudberg MA, Brody JA. Gastrostomy placement and mortality among hospitalized Medicare beneficiaries. JAMA 1998;279:1973–6.
6. Kurien M, Leeds JS, Delegge MH, et al. Mortality among patients who receive or defer gastrostomies. Clin Gastroenterol Hepatol 2013;11:1445–50.
7. Larson DE, Burton DD, Schroeder KW, et al. Percutaneous endoscopic gastrostomy. Indications, success, complications, and mortality in 314 consecutive patients. Gastroenterology 1987;93:48–52.
8. Hull MA, Rawlings J, Field J, et al. Audit of outcome of long-term enteral nutrition by percutaneous endoscopic gastrostomy. Lancet 1993;341(8849):869–72.
9. Mathus-Vliegen LM, Koning H. Percutaneous endoscopic gastrostomy and gastrojejunostomy: a critical reappraisal of patient selection, tube function and the feasibility of nutritional support during extended follow-up. Gastrointest Endosc 1999;50:746–54.
10. Schneider AS, Schettler A, Markowski A, et al. Complication and mortality rate after percutaneous endoscopic gastrostomy are low and indication-dependent. Scand J Gastroenterol 2014;49:891–8.
11. Gottfried EB, Plumser AB, Clair MR. Pneumoperitoneum following percutaneous endoscopic gastrostomy. A prospective study. Gastrointest Endosc 1986;32: 397–9.
12. Wojtowycz MM, Arata JA Jr, Micklos TJ, et al. CT findings after uncomplicated percutaneous gastrostomy. Am J Roentgenol 1988;151:307–9.
13. Wiesen AJ, Sideridis K, Fernandes A, et al. True incidence and clinical significance of pneumoperitoneum after PEG placement: a prospective study. Gastrointest Endosc 2006;64:886–9.

14. Blum CA, Selander C, Ruddy JM, et al. The incidence and clinical significance of pneumoperitoneum after percutaneous endoscopic gastrostomy: a review of 722 cases. Am Surg 2009;75:39–43.
15. Shah RD, Tariq N, Shanley C, et al. Peritonitis from peg tube insertion in surgical intensive care unit patients: identification of risk factors and clinical outcomes. Surg Endosc 2009;23:2580–6.
16. Nishiwaki S, Araki H, Hayashi M, et al. Inhibitory effects of carbon dioxide insufflation on pneumoperitoneum and bowel distension after percutaneous endoscopic gastrostomy. World J Gastroenterol 2012;18:3565–70.
17. Kirby DF, DeLegge MH, Fleming CR. American Gastroenterological Association technical review on tube feeding for enteral nutrition. Gastroenterology 1995; 108:1282–301.
18. Kitamura T, Nakase H, Iizuka H. Risk factors for aspiration pneumonia after percutaneous endoscopic gastrostomy. Gerontology 2007;53:224–7.
19. Finucane TE, Christmas C, Travis K. Tube feeding in patients with advanced dementia: a review of the evidence. JAMA 1999;282:1365–70.
20. Dharmarajan TS, Yadav D, Adiga GU, et al. Gastrostomy, esophagitis, and gastrointestinal bleeding in older adults. J Am Med Dir Assoc 2004;5:228–32.
21. Ahmad J, Thomson S, McFall B, et al. Colonic injury following percutaneous endoscopic-guided gastrostomy insertion. BMJ Case Rep 2010;2010. pii: bcr0520102976.
22. Guloglu R, Taviloglu K, Alimoglu O. Colon injury following percutaneous endoscopic gastrostomy tube insertion. J Laparoendosc Adv Surg Tech A 2003;13: 69–72.
23. Wiggins TF, Kaplan R, DeLegge MH. Acute hemorrhage following transhepatic PEG tube placement. Dig Dis Sci 2007;52:167–9.
24. Gubler C, Wildi SM, Bauerfeind P. Liver injury during PEG tube placement: report of two cases. Gastrointest Endosc 2005;61:346–8.
25. Chaer RA, Rekkas D, Trevino J, et al. Intrahepatic placement of a PEG tube. Gastrointest Endosc 2003;57:763–5.
26. Richter JA, Patrie JT, Richter RP, et al. Bleeding after percutaneous endoscopic gastrostomy is linked to serotonin reuptake inhibitors, not aspirin or clopidogrel. Gastrointest Endosc 2011;74:22–34.
27. Singh D, Laya AS, Vaidya OU, et al. Risk of bleeding after percutaneous endoscopic gastrostomy (PEG). Dig Dis Sci 2011;57:973–80.
28. Lau G, Lai SH. Fatal retroperitoneal haemorrhage: an unusual complication of percutaneous endoscopic gastrostomy. Forensic Sci Int 2001;116:69–75.
29. ASGE Standards of Practice Committee, Anderson MA, Ben-Menachem T, et al. Management of antithrombotic agents for endoscopic procedures. Gastrointest Endosc 2009;70:1060–70.
30. Nishiwaki S, Araki H, Takada J, et al. Clinical investigation of upper gastrointestinal hemorrhage after percutaneous endoscopic gastrostomy. Dig Endosc 2010;22:180–5.
31. Lockett MA, Templeton ML, Byrne TK, et al. Percutaneous endoscopic gastrostomy complications in a tertiary-care center. Am Surg 2002;68:117–20.
32. Ahmad I, Mouncher A, Abdoolah A, et al. Antibiotic prophylaxis for percutaneous endoscopic gastrostomy: a prospective, randomised, double-blind trial. Aliment Pharmacol Ther 2003;18:209–15.
33. Jafri NS, Mahid SS, Minor KS, et al. Meta-analysis: antibiotic prophylaxis to prevent peristomal infection following percutaneous endoscopic gastrostomy. Aliment Pharmacol Ther 2007;25:647–56.

34. ASGE Standards of Practice Committee, Banerjee S, Shen B, et al. Antibiotic prophylaxis for GI endoscopy. Gastrointest Endosc 2008;67:791–8.
35. Thomas S, Cantrill S, Waghorn DJ, et al. The role of screening and antibiotic prophylaxis in the prevention of percutaneous gastrostomy site infection caused by methicillin-resistant *Staphylococcus aureus*. Aliment Pharmacol Ther 2007;25: 593–7.
36. Cave DR, Robinson WR, Brotschi EA. Necrotizing fasciitis following percutaneous endoscopic gastrostomy. Gastrointest Endosc 1986;32:294–6.
37. Greif JM, Ragland JJ, Ochsner MG, et al. Fatal necrotizing fasciitis complicating percutaneous endoscopic gastrostomy. Gastrointest Endosc 1986;32:292–4.
38. Person JL, Brower RA. Necrotizing fasciitis/myositis following percutaneous endoscopic gastrostomy. Gastrointest Endosc 1986;32:309.
39. Wirth R, Bauer J, Sieber C. Necrotizing *Candida* infection after percutaneous endoscopic gastrostomy: a fatal and rare complication. JPEN J Parenter Enteral Nutr 2008;32:285–7.
40. Martindale R, Witte M, Hodges G, et al. Necrotizing fasciitis as a complication of percutaneous endoscopic gastrostomy. JPEN J Parenter Enteral Nutr 1987;11: 583–5.
41. Pop GH. Buried bumper syndrome: can we prevent it? Pract Gastroenterol 2010; 34(5):8–13.
42. Gencosmanoglu R, Koc D, Tozun N. The buried bumper syndrome: migration of internal bumper of percutaneous endoscopic gastrostomy tube into the abdominal wall. J Gastroenterol 2003;38:1077–80.
43. Tsai J, Lin H. Clinical manifestations and management of buried bumper syndrome in patients with percutaneous endoscopic gastrostomy. Gastrointest Endosc 2009;69:1193–4.
44. Christiaens P, Bossuyt P, Cuyle PJ, et al. Buried bumper syndrome: single-step endoscopic management and replacement. Gastrointest Endosc 2014;80(2):336.
45. Braden B, Brandstaetter M, Caspary WF, et al. Buried bumper syndrome: treatment guided by catheter probe US. Gastrointest Endosc 2003;57:747–51.
46. Okutani D, Kotani K, Makihara S. A case of gastrocolocutaneous fistula as a complication of percutaneous endoscopic gastrostomy. Acta Med Okayama 2008;62:135–8.
47. Mollitt DL, Dokler ML, Evans JS, et al. Complications of retained internal bolster after pediatric percutaneous endoscopic gastrostomy. J Pediatr Surg 1998;33:271–3.
48. Date RS, Das A, Bateson PG. Unusual complications of ballooned feeding tubes. Ir Med J 2002;95:181–2.
49. Chong VH. Gastric outlet obstruction caused by gastrostomy tube balloon. Indian J Gastroenterol 2004;23:80–2.
50. Fischer LS, Bonello JC, Greenberg E. Gastrostomy tube migration and gastric outlet obstruction following percutaneous endoscopic gastrostomy. Gastrointest Endosc 1987;33:381–2.
51. Galea MH, Mayell MJ. Gastroduodenal mucosal intussusception causing gastric outlet obstruction: a complication of gastrostomy tubes. J Pediatr Surg 1988;23: 980–1.
52. Oswald MP, Graviss ER, Danis RK, et al. Duodenogastric intussusception causing gastric outlet obstruction. J Pediatr Surg 1982;17:82–3.
53. Cappell MS. Risk factors and risk reduction of malignant seeding of the percutaneous endoscopic gastrostomy track from pharyngoesophageal malignancy: a review of all 44 known reported cases. Am J Gastroenterol 2007; 102:1307–11.

54. Cruz I, Mamel JJ, Brady PG, et al. Incidence of abdominal wall metastasis complicating PEG tube placement in untreated head and neck cancer. Gastrointest Endosc 2005;62(5):708–11.

55. Douglas JG, Koh WJ, Laramore GE. Metastasis to a percutaneous gastrostomy site from head and neck cancer: radiobiologic considerations. Head Neck 2000;22:826–30.

56. Yoskovitch A, Hier MP, Okrainec A, et al. Skin metastases in squamous cell carcinoma of the head and neck. Otolaryngol Head Neck Surg 2001;124:248–52.

57. Pickhardt PJ, Charles A, Rohrmann J, et al. Stomal metastases complicating percutaneous endoscopic gastrostomy: CT findings and the argument for radiologic tube placement. Am J Roentgenol 2002;179:735–9.

58. Rosenberger LH, Newhook T, Schirmer B, et al. Late accidental dislodgement of a percutaneous endoscopic gastrostomy tube: an underestimated burden on patients and the health care system. Surg Endosc 2011;25:3307–11.

59. Wu FY, Wu JF, Ni YH. Long-term outcome after percutaneous endoscopic gastrostomy in children. Pediatr Neonatol 2013;54:326–9.

60. Panagiotakis PH, DiSario JA, Hilden K, et al. DPEJ tube placement prevents aspiration pneumonia in high-risk patients. Nutr Clin Pract 2008;23:172–5.

61. Fan AC, Baron TH, Rumalla A, et al. Comparison of direct percutaneous endoscopic jejunostomy and PEG with jejunal extension. Gastrointest Endosc 2002; 56:890–4.

62. Maple JT, Petersen BT, Baron TH, et al. Direct percutaneous endoscopic jejunostomy: outcomes in 307 consecutive attempts. Am J Gastroenterol 2005;100: 2681–8.

Complications of Enteroscopy: How to Avoid Them and Manage Them When They Arise

CrossMark

Disaya Chavalitdhamrong, MD[a], Douglas G. Adler, MD[b], Peter V. Draganov, MD[a],*

KEYWORDS

- Enteroscopy • Small bowel endoscopy • Double-balloon enteroscopy
- Single-balloon enteroscopy • Spiral enteroscopy • Adverse events • Perforation
- Pancreatitis

KEY POINTS

- Deep small bowel enteroscopy is a safe procedure, but enteroscopy-associated adverse events are more common compared with standard endoscopy.
- The 2 most common serious adverse events are perforation and pancreatitis.
- Familiarity with the technical aspects of deep small bowel enteroscopy, careful performance, and awareness of the potential adverse event are the key to successful and safe procedure.

INTRODUCTION

The small bowel has remained the final frontier for endoscopic exploration of the luminal gastrointestinal (GI) tract. Over the last decade, deep small bowel enteroscopy has dramatically improved and has now moved into the realm of routine gastroenterology practice. This progress had led to a significant improvement in the diagnostic capabilities and treatment strategies available to the patient. Although enteroscopy is generally a safe procedure, the rate of adverse events is higher than conventional upper or lower endoscopy. Knowledge of potential endoscopic adverse events, their expected frequency, and the risk factors associated with their occurrence may help to minimize the incidence of adverse events.

The authors have no conflicts of interest to disclose.

[a] Division of Gastroenterology, Hepatology and Nutrition, Department of Internal Medicine, University of Florida, Gainesville, FL, USA; [b] Division of Gastroenterology and Hepatology, Department of Internal Medicine, University of Utah School of Medicine, 30 North 1900 East 4R 118, Salt Lake City, UT 84132, USA

* Corresponding author. Division of Gastroenterology, Hepatology and Nutrition, Department of Internal Medicine, University of Florida, 1329 Southwest 16th Street, Suite 5251, Gainesville, FL 32608.

E-mail address: dragapv@medicine.ufl.edu

Gastrointest Endoscopy Clin N Am 25 (2015) 83–95
http://dx.doi.org/10.1016/j.giec.2014.09.002
1052-5157/15/$ – see front matter Published by Elsevier Inc.

TYPES OF DEEP SMALL BOWEL ENTEROSCOPY PROCEDURES

There are 3 deep small bowel enteroscopy platforms referred to as overtube-assisted or device-assisted deep small bowel enteroscopy. These platforms include double-balloon enteroscopy (DBE), single-balloon enteroscopy (SBE), and spiral enteroscopy. All 3 systems are comparable regarding insertion depths, diagnostic and therapeutic efficacies, and adverse event rates. The choice of enteroscopy technique depends on availability, personal experience, and clinical implication. All enteroscopy platforms can be used in antegrade (per oral) or retrograde (per rectum) routes. The depth of insertion by antegrade route is about 200 to 250 cm beyond the ligament of Treitz. Enteroscopy via the antegrade route has been reported to have a higher diagnostic and therapeutic yield as well as higher success rate and faster learning curve than the retrograde route.[1,2] In some cases, the entire small bowel can be evaluated using a combination of antegrade and retrograde approaches (also known as total entero-scopy), but this cannot be reliably and routinely accomplished in all patients.[3–5]

Both DBE and SBE (also known as balloon-assisted enteroscopy) consist of a 200-cm working length enteroscope and a 140-cm to 145-cm soft overtube. Tech-nique for advancement uses a push and pull method, with inflation and deflation of the balloon(s) and telescoping of the small intestine onto the overtube. This telescoping allows the endoscope to advance a longer distance compared with con-ventional push enteroscopy with minimal looping. Every 5 cm of overtube advance-ment resembles 40 cm of small bowel visualized. DBE is the most frequently enteroscopy platform used, because it was introduced first in 2001 and has relatively high rates of total enteroscopy (>40%). The system uses 2 types of endoscopes (reg-ular or therapeutic scope). SBE was introduced in 2007. It seems that total entero-scopy is more easily performed and achieved with DBE than with SBE; however, diagnostic yield and adverse event rate are comparable.[6–8]

Spiral enteroscopy is the most recently introduced technique, in which an endo-scope is fitted with a rotating overtube that has a soft spiral fin at the tip.[9] Spiral entero-scopy involves the rotation of a spiral-tipped overtube device, thus, pleating the small bowel to allow deep small bowel evaluation and interventions. Retrograde spiral enteroscopy is usually needed to achieve total enteroscopy, if at all.[10] Spiral entero-scopy has been reported to be as safe as DBE, with similar diagnostic and therapeutic yield,[11] but it involves shorter examination times.[12] It also allows the enteroscope to be removed and reintroduced while holding the position deep in the small bowel using the spiral overtube. This technique can be particularly useful when multiple polypectomies are required in patients with intestinal polyposis syndromes such as Peutz-Jeghers syndrome.

INDICATIONS FOR ENTEROSCOPY

The indications for enteroscopy include diagnosis and therapeutic interventions for small intestinal diseases and have continued to expand. Because the rate of adverse events related to enteroscopy is higher than conventional upper or lower endoscopy, a well-established indication is strongly endorsed. The most common indication for enteroscopy is the evaluation and diagnosis of small bowel lesions as a cause of iron deficiency anemia, GI bleeding, and suspected inflammatory bowel disease or mass. Enteroscopy-guided therapy in patients with obscure GI bleeding is cost effective and has been shown to reduce the rate of overt bleeding and the need for iron supplementation, blood transfusions, and additional invasive proce-dures.[13–16] Additional indications include retrieving retained video capsules and biopsy/marking of lesions for further laparoscopic management.[17] Enteroscopy can also be used in patients with surgically altered upper GI anatomy, such as Roux-en-Y gastric bypass, to examine the excluded segment of the small bowel or excluded gastric remnant and also as a platform for endoscopic retrograde cholangiopancreatography (ERCP).[18,19] Recently, deep small bowel enteroscopy endoscopes have been shown to be a useful tool in patients with difficult colonoscopy and failed colonoscopy.[20] Reported indications for deep small bowel enteroscopy along with diagnostic and therapeutic maneuvers are summarized in **Box 1**.

Box 1
Reported indications and diagnostic/therapeutic interventions of enteroscopy

Reported indications

- Obscure GI bleeding (overt and occult)
- Chronic diarrhea
- Iron deficiency anemia
- Celiac disease
- Small bowel Crohn disease
- Small bowel fistula
- Small bowel tumors
- Anastomotic stricture or evaluation of an anastomosis
- History of intestinal polyps (familial adenomatous polyposis, Gardner, Peutz-Jeghers)
- Abnormal capsule endoscopy or other radiographic imaging study
- Therapeutic ERCP in patients with altered upper GI anatomy

Reported diagnostic and therapeutic interventions

- Luminal
  - Hemostasis (injection, argon plasma, and bipolar coagulation)
  - Biopsy
  - Polypectomy
  - Stricture dilation
  - Enteral stent placement
  - Percutaneous endoscopic jejunostomy tube placement
  - Percutaneous endoscopic gastrostomy tube placement in the excluded stomach in Roux-en-Y gastric bypass patients
  - Fistula plug placement, fistula closure using clips and loops
  - Foreign body retrieval (retained video capsule, percutaneous endoscopic gastrostomy tube bumper, gastric balloon in the jejunum, impacted esophageal stent in the ileum, migrated biliary stent in the distal ileum)
  - India ink tattoo
- Pancreaticobiliary
  - Cannulation/sphincterotomy/balloon sphincteroplasty
  - Stone/sludge extraction
  - Stent placement/removal
  - Stricture dilation

The need for routine use of capsule endoscopy or other small bowel imaging study before enteroscopy remains a controversial issue. Prescreening patients with capsule endoscopy improves the diagnostic and therapeutic yield of enteroscopy.[21] Preferential use of capsule endoscopy followed by enteroscopy for obscure GI bleeding has been suggested as a diagnostic strategy.[22] The use of capsule endoscopy before enteroscopy has also been shown to be cost effective for diagnosis and possible therapeutic interventions in small bowel Crohn disease.[23] Furthermore, capsule endoscopy is safe, and adverse events are uncommon. On the other hand, capsule endoscopy and other small bowel imaging studies are frequently nondiagnostic and do not provide any therapeutic capabilities. Therefore, capsule endoscopy before enteroscopy should not be performed routinely, but on a case-by-case basis.

CONTRAINDICATIONS

Enteroscopy can be safely performed in most patients. DBE has a high and increasing diagnostic yield with age, leading to a high positive impact on management in elderly patients.[24–26] DBE has also been reported as a safe tool in children.[27] Furthermore, DBE has also been reported to be equally safe and effective when performed in a community setting compared with a tertiary referral center with a comparable yield, efficacy, and adverse event rate.[28] In addition, the diagnostic and therapeutic yields are not influenced by the timing of enteroscopy (morning vs afternoon).[29]

Patients with suspected or impending GI perforation should not undergo enteroscopy. If deep enteroscopy is required with a true latex allergy, SBE or spiral enteroscopy should be considered, because the DBE balloons contain latex.[30]

Overtube-assisted enteroscopy is relatively contraindicated in patients with esophageal stricture or varices. Spiral enteroscopy in particular should be avoided in these patients because the spiral overtube has a larger diameter compared with DBE and SBE. Moreover, the overtubes used with DBE and SBE do not require mechanical rotation and may be a safer choice. However, in the absence of robust comparative data, there are no specific guidelines as to which enteroscopy platform to use in particular clinical situations, and decisions must be individualized to each patient and condition.

GENERAL RULES OF THUMB

There are various technical aspects in performing deep small bowel enteroscopy with the different platforms, but some general rules of thumb apply:

- Enteroscopy performed in appropriately selected individuals is a highly useful and safe clinical tool. Select patients carefully to maximize procedural efficacy, safety and minimize its adverse events.
- Review clinical data, including medications, carefully and identify high-risk patients for proper plans on type of sedation, endoscopic option, interventions, and so forth.
- A well-defined indication is required before performing enteroscopy. Review of all previous studies, including radiologic small bowel imaging and capsule endoscopy findings, is imperative for estimating the approximate location of a lesion and planning an antegrade versus retrograde approach. Review of previous surgeries to understand the patient's altered GI altered anatomy is also essential for preprocedural considerations.
- Carefully select the anticoagulation and antiplatelet management options. If a decision is made to perform endoscopy in patients receiving antithrombotic

therapy, the need to stop or reverse these agents should be individualized.[31] Performing the procedure while continuing these agents may be associated with higher yield in bleeding cases. No prospective data are available to determine which international normalized ratio is necessary for endoscopic therapy to be safe and effective. Several new anticoagulants and antiplatelet agents were recently approved, and their use as it relates to endoscopy was summarized in a recent review.[32] Endoscopists should be familiar with these medications to optimize outcomes and seek input of relevant consultants (eg, cardiology, hematology, and neurology) before discontinuing any antithrombotic agents.

- Careful enteroscope insertion, examination, and intervention are essential to avoid adverse events. The guiding principle while performing deep small bowel enteroscopy should be to be gentle. This principle should be kept in mind for careful performance of enteroscopy, especially with deep sedation delivered by an anesthesiologist. Perform enteroscopy with extra care in high-risk patients/procedures.

- Look for disease on the way in and look for trauma on the way out on DBE and SBE, but look for both disease and trauma on the way out on spiral enteroscopy, because collapsed lumen is needed for pleating the small bowel while advancing the scope, which significantly impairs visualization.

- Carbon dioxide insufflation is preferred for enteroscopy, because of its rapid absorption and should be used if available. Significantly less gas is retained in the small bowel with carbon dioxide use compared with air insufflation.[32] Furthermore, during DBE, fewer patients had severe pain with carbon dioxide than with air insufflation.[33,34] No significant difference in pre-DBE and post-DBE partial pressure of oxygen in the blood and partial pressure of carbon dioxide in the blood was noted between the 2 groups. Although data have supported the safety and efficacy of carbon dioxide insufflation for endoscopy, most studies excluded patients with severe respiratory compromise or chronic obstructive pulmonary disease. Therefore, it would be prudent to consider room air insufflation in those who are potentially at risk for ventilatory compromise with carbon dioxide insufflation until the question is further studied.

- Fluoroscopy can be helpful in providing information such as the scope tip position, scope tip movement, loop information, and guidance for loop reduction. However, routine use of fluoroscopy is not needed particularly with more experienced operators, although if available its use should be considered.

- It is important to be aware of one's own level of experience and available support. Studies reported that antegrade SBE has a faster learning curve than the retrograde route. Twenty to 35 cases of retrograde DBE are typically needed before achieving stable overtube intubation of the ileum.[1,35,36] In addition, significant decrease in overall procedural and fluoroscopy time has been shown after the initial 10 antegrade DBE, whereas there was no change in timing for retrograde DBE.[37]

- An experienced enteroscopy team is essential. The enteroscopy team should be familiar with all the steps involved in these complex multistage procedures to avoid confusion and ensure success.[36,38] DBE requires the repetition of a series of multiple maneuvers (inflating/deflating the scope and overtube balloons, advancing/reducing the scope, advancing/reducing the overtube). Therefore, confusion can easily occur, and valuable time can be wasted figuring out the correct stage of the procedure. Furthermore, pushing/pulling the scope/overtube with the wrong inflated balloon can contribute to adverse events. The SBE platform has only 1 balloon and requires fewer stages but nevertheless losing track of the proper maneuver sequence can easily occur. Spiral enteroscopy requires the active hands-on involvement of an assistant to rotate clockwise/counterclockwise and pull/push the spiral overtube. These maneuvers have to be coordinated with the enteroscope steering and advancement/shortening while the overtube is coupled or uncoupled from the scope. All deep enteroscopy procedures require an experienced team with a high degree of coordination.

- It is necessary to be fully aware of particular potential enteroscopy-related adverse events to avoid these events from occurring.

ADVERSE EVENTS

The potential adverse events of enteroscopy are summarized in **Box 2**. The reported incidence of adverse events for the 3 deep small bowel enteroscopy platforms is shown in **Table 1**.

Common or Major Adverse Events

The adverse event rate with enteroscopy is higher compared with that associated with conventional GI endoscopy.[39] Enteroscopy also has the potential for unique adverse events, such as acute pancreatitis associated with all enteroscopy systems and esophageal mucosal trauma associated mostly with spiral enteroscopy.[40] Adverse events can be related to diagnostic procedure and therapeutic interventions. Most data are from DBE studies. The adverse event rate has been reported to be between 0.7% and 20% with major adverse events rate in approximately 1% of diagnostic procedures and 2.3% to 5% of therapeutic procedures.[5,14,24,41–45] The incidence of adverse events seems comparable among all device-assisted enteroscopy platforms.[46] Sore throat, intussusception, abdominal distention, and self-limited abdominal pain have been reported in as many as 20% of patients.[4,47] Common and major

---

Box 2
Reported adverse events of enteroscopy

Reported common and major adverse events

- GI bleeding
- Mucosal injury
- Perforation
- Acute pancreatitis
- Hyperamylasemia
- Sedation-related complications
- Intussusception, sore throat, abdominal distention, and abdominal pain

Rarely reported and minor adverse events

- Intestinal necrosis
- Subcutaneous emphysema
- Transient pneumobilia
- Intraperitoneal bleeding
- Superior mesenteric vein thrombosis

Table 1
Overview of enteroscopy adverse events

Technique	Adverse Event	Rate (%)
DBE	Overall	0.3–5[1]
	Perforation (overall)	1.2[48]
	Perforation (with therapeutic interventions)	6.5[45]
	Bleeding (with therapeutic interventions)	4.3[45]
	Acute pancreatitis	0.3–1[48,57]
	Hyperamylasemia	17–51[57,68,69]
	Minor complications/discomfort	20[47]
SBE	Overall	0.6–3.8[46,70]
Spiral enteroscopy	Overall	0.031–28
	Minor complications/discomfort	19–28[71]
	Pinch/torque injury	0.031–22[52,59]
	Perforation	0.34[72]

adverse events include GI bleeding, perforation, acute pancreatitis, and sedation-related adverse events.[48]

Bleeding can be from mucosal tear, partially treated bleeding lesions such as arteriovenous malformations, esophageal varices, or an adverse event of therapeutic intervention, such as polypectomy and stricture dilation. Mucosal trauma can occur to esophagus, stomach, small bowel, and colon. Mucosal injury is more common with spiral enteroscopy, especially to the esophageal mucosa. Partial-thickness tears or mucosal disruptions occurred in 3 of 78 patients undergoing antegrade spiral entero-scopy procedures (2 in the esophagus, 1 in the prepyloric region).[15] No complete perforations occurred. The prepyloric region was treated with endoclips, and the other 2 required no further therapy.

Perforation can occur at the anastomotic site, in the deep small bowel, or at other weak points in the small bowel. Perforation may also occur in altered anatomy because of fixation of the bowel from adhesions and resultant tearing. Stalling of enteroscope passage because of bowel fixation should alert the endoscopist to this later possibility. Endoscopists may not be aware of the perforation if it occurs at a site proximal to the scope tip. Delayed perforation can be seen as a result of thermal injury. The reported perforation rate varies from less than 1% to as high as 6.5% and seems higher in patients undergoing therapeutic enteroscopy, especially polypec-tomy of large polyps and in patients with altered surgical anatomy undergoing retro-grade procedure.[8,45,49]

Acute pancreatitis is a particular adverse event related to enteroscopy. The rate of acute pancreatitis has been reported to be between 0.3% and 1%.[4,5,41,43,48,50] Acute pancreatitis is mainly an adverse event of antegrade enteroscopy, with only 1 case after retrograde DBE.[51,52] The severity has been reported as mild to moderate. The causal mechanism of acute pancreatitis is uncertain.[50] Postulated mechanisms for the development of acute pancreatitis caused by enteroscopy are an increase in duodenal intraluminal pressure during the procedure, which leads the reflux of duodenal fluids into the pancreatic duct,[53] or mechanical straining of the endoscope with overtube (by scope, overtube, or balloon) on the pancreas or in the ampullary area.[50] There are no effective prophylactic maneuvers.

Hyperamylasemia is frequently observed after antegrade enteroscopy but often without associated pancreatitis.[54] Hyperamylasemia could be related to focal points of pancreatic ischemia caused by mechanical stress as well as mechanical trauma to the mesentery.[55] Hyperamylasemia can also originate from salivary amylasemia.[56] The incidence of hyperamylasemia has been reported in up to 51% of patients undergoing enteroscopy and seems to be associated with longer procedure time and insertion depth.[57] A possible preventive strategy that can be applied at the time of DBE is to reduce the time between the first and second inflations of the overtube balloon.[58] A long time between 2 inflations might act as a mechanical stress factor related to more enteroscope movement or more air insufflation.

Sedation-related adverse events include hypotension, oxygen desaturation/hypoxia, hypoventilation, bradycardia, hypertension, arrhythmia, aspiration, and allergic reactions. Enteroscopy can be successfully and safely accomplished with moderate (conscious) sedation, but general anesthesia is preferred for a longer procedure to protect the airway form aspiration.[59] Respiratory compromise can be an issue, because enteroscope withdrawal by unpleating bowel takes time and rapid withdrawal can cause intussusception, so general anesthesia with tracheal intubation may be required in high-risk patients. No direct comparative studies are available, but many centers in the United States perform deep small bowel enteroscopy exclusively under general anesthesia with endotracheal intubation.

Rarely Reported Adverse Events

Intestinal necrosis at the epinephrine injection site after DBE procedure has been reported.[60] The patient experienced bleeding 2 days after the procedure. Surgical resection showed ischemic necrosis at the injection site for presumed bleeding of an angiodysplastic lesion in the jejunum. The injection was with a total of 3 mL of 1 in 10,000 epinephrine in hypertonic saline. The investigators discussed that the thinner wall of the small intestine may be the cause of adverse events. Reported risk factors for intestinal necrosis after epinephrine injection are advanced age, atherosclerotic vascular disease, anemia, hypoxemia, and shock.[61]

Subcutaneous emphysema without a visible intestinal perforation after a retrograde DBE has occurred.[62] The investigators commented that the prolonged duration of the procedure and overtube balloon use caused high-pressure air to diffuse to the retroperitoneum. Existing ileal inflammation may also have augmented the air diffusion.

A case of transient pneumobilia after DBE with balloon dilation for strictures of Crohn disease has been reported.[63] It was detected during the procedure without any symptoms. The investigators suggested that the increased duodenal air pressure from enteroscopy may have induced transient incompetence of the sphincter of Oddi. The frequency of pneumobilia after enteroscopy is unknown and may be underestimated because of the lack of symptoms. Use of carbon dioxide insufflation can reduce this adverse event, given its rapid absorption. The mechanism of this adverse event might be similar to more serious adverse events, such as air embolism. In 1 report[64] of a patient who had had Whipple surgery and underwent ERCP, the patient developed embolic infarctions of cerebrum and spinal cord, causing stroke with paraplegia. Using carbon dioxide insufflation was recommended to avoid/alleviate these adverse events.

Two cases of intraperitoneal bleeding related to enteroscopy have been described. The first case was after an antegrade DBE, without any obvious small bowel trauma during the procedure.[65] This adverse event occurred in a patient who had undergone a small bowel resection 3 years earlier. In patients with previous abdominal surgery who experience abdominal pain and decreased hemoglobin levels after enteroscopy, intraperitoneal bleeding should be included as a potential adverse event. A second case of intraperitoneal bleeding was associated with spiral enteroscopy in a patient who had undergone left nephrectomy.[66] Previous intra-abdominal surgery is the major risk factor for this adverse event. Enteroscopy can compress, stretch, and shear adhesions and the mesentery, with the potential of disruption of blood vessels.

Superior mesenteric artery thrombosis related to DBE in a patient with Crohn disease has been recognized.[67]

MANAGEMENT STRATEGIES

The lack of a universally accepted management strategy of enteroscopy-associated adverse events relates to the small sample size of available studies. The following points are based on the available data and the authors' experience.

- Awareness and early recognition of adverse events are essential.
- Small bowel intussusception typically resolves spontaneously, but careful observation of the patient is needed.
- Endoscopic treatment of perforation and bleeding should be considered first.
- If perforation is discovered immediately, endoscopic therapy is preferred (ie, using traditional clip, over the scope clip, or suturing device). It is important to be cognizant which closure device can operate with a particular endoscope (eg, the endoscopic suturing device cannot be used with the enteroscope, and exchange to the double-channel upper endoscope is needed if the perforation is in the reach of the upper scope). If overt perforation is not amenable to endoscopic therapy, surgery is needed. If perforation is delayed, computed tomography imaging is needed to define extraluminal fluid collections. Surgery with drainage of fluid collections is needed with delayed perforation.
- Endoscopic treatment of bleeding is typically first considered using the traditional endoscopic therapies, including injection therapy, thermal coagulation, hemostatic clips, argon plasma coagulation, and combination therapy.
- Hyperamylasemia is frequently observed after deep enteroscopy but often without associated pancreatitis. Thus, treatment is generally not required.
- Management of enteroscopy-related pancreatitis is similar to that of acute pancreatitis caused by other causes. Enteroscopy-related pancreatitis is usually not severe, although cases of necrotizing pancreatitis and death have been described.[50]

SUMMARY

Enteroscopy has transformed the management of small bowel diseases. It is a safe procedure with an acceptable adverse event rate, but adverse events do occur at a higher rate than with standard upper and lower endoscopy. However, endoscopists performing enteroscopy should be aware that these events can occur and may have delayed presentations. Knowledge of potential endoscopic adverse events, their expected frequency, and the risk factors for their occurrence may help to minimize their incidence. Endoscopists are expected to carefully select patients, have familiarity with the planned procedure and available technology, and be prepared to manage any adverse events that may arise. Once an adverse event occurs, early recognition and prompt intervention minimize the morbidity and mortality associated with that adverse event.

REFERENCES

1. Dutta AK, Sajith KG, Joseph AJ, et al. Learning curve, diagnostic yield and safety of single balloon enteroscopy. Trop Gastroenterol 2012;33(3):179–84.

2. Sanaka MR, Navaneethan U, Kosuru B, et al. Antegrade is more effective than retrograde enteroscopy for evaluation and management of suspected small-bowel disease. Clin Gastroenterol Hepatol 2012;10(8):910–6.

3. Yamamoto H, Sekine Y, Sato Y, et al. Total enteroscopy with a nonsurgical steerable double-balloon method. Gastrointest Endosc 2001;53(2):216–20.

4. Heine GD, Hadithi M, Groenen MJ, et al. Double-balloon enteroscopy: indications, diagnostic yield, and complications in a series of 275 patients with suspected small-bowel disease. Endoscopy 2006;38(1):42–8.

5. Xin L, Liao Z, Jiang YP, et al. Indications, detectability, positive findings, total enteroscopy, and complications of diagnostic double-balloon endoscopy: a systematic review of data over the first decade of use. Gastrointest Endosc 2011;74(3):563–70.

6. Kawamura T, Yasuda K, Tanaka K, et al. Clinical evaluation of a newly developed single-balloon enteroscope. Gastrointest Endosc 2008;68(6):1112–6.

7. Takano N, Yamada A, Watabe H, et al. Single-balloon versus double-balloon endoscopy for achieving total enteroscopy: a randomized, controlled trial. Gastrointest Endosc 2011;73(4):734–9.

8. Gerson LB. Capsule endoscopy and deep enteroscopy. Gastrointest Endosc 2013;78(3):439–43.

9. Yamada A, Watabe H, Oka S, et al. Feasibility of spiral enteroscopy in Japanese patients: study in two tertiary hospitals. Dig Endosc 2013;25(4):406–11.

10. Nagula S, Gaidos J, Draganov PV, et al. Retrograde spiral enteroscopy: feasibility, success, and safety in a series of 22 patients. Gastrointest Endosc 2011; 74(3):699–702.

11. Rahmi G, Samaha E, Vahedi K, et al. Multicenter comparison of double-balloon enteroscopy and spiral enteroscopy. J Gastroenterol Hepatol 2013;28(6): 992–8.

12. Messer I, May A, Manner H, et al. Prospective, randomized, single-center trial comparing double-balloon enteroscopy and spiral enteroscopy in patients with suspected small-bowel disorders. Gastrointest Endosc 2013;77(2):241–9.

13. Lin WP, Chiu CT, Su MY, et al. Treatment decision for potential bleeders in obscure gastrointestinal bleeding during double-balloon enteroscopy. Dig Dis Sci 2009;54(10):2192–7.

14. Samaha E, Rahmi G, Landi B, et al. Long-term outcome of patients treated with double balloon enteroscopy for small bowel vascular lesions. Am J Gastroenterol 2012;107(2):240–6.

15. Williamson JB, Judah JR, Gaidos JK, et al. Prospective evaluation of the long-term outcomes after deep small-bowel spiral enteroscopy in patients with obscure GI bleeding. Gastrointest Endosc 2012;76(4):771–8.

16. Shishido T, Oka S, Tanaka S, et al. Outcome of patients who have undergone total enteroscopy for obscure gastrointestinal bleeding. World J Gastroenterol 2012; 18(7):666–72.

17. Roorda AK, Kupec JT, Ostrinsky Y, et al. Endoscopic approach to capsule endoscope retention. Expert Rev Gastroenterol Hepatol 2010;4(6):713–21.

18. Patel MK, Horsley-Silva JL, Gomez V, et al. Double balloon enteroscopy procedure in patients with surgically altered bowel anatomy: analysis of a large prospectively collected database. J Laparoendosc Adv Surg Tech A 2013; 23(5):409–13.

19. Wagh MS, Draganov PV. Prospective evaluation of spiral overtube-assisted ERCP in patients with surgically altered anatomy. Gastrointest Endosc 2012;76(2): 439–43.

20. Yamada A, Watabe H, Takano N, et al. Utility of single and double balloon endoscopy in patients with difficult colonoscopy: a randomized controlled trial. World J Gastroenterol 2013;19(29):4732–6.

21. Sethi S, Cohen J, Thaker AM, et al. Prior capsule endoscopy improves the diagnostic and therapeutic yield of single-balloon enteroscopy. Dig Dis Sci 2014;59:2497–502.

22. Shishido T, Oka S, Tanaka S, et al. Diagnostic yield of capsule endoscopy vs. double-balloon endoscopy for patients who have undergone total enteroscopy with obscure gastrointestinal bleeding. Hepatogastroenterology 2012;59(116): 955–9.

23. Tharian B, Caddy G, Tham TC. Enteroscopy in small bowel Crohn's disease: a review. World J Gastrointest Endosc 2013;5(10):476–86.

24. Hegde SR, Iffrig K, Li T, et al. Double-balloon enteroscopy in the elderly: safety, findings, and diagnostic and therapeutic success. Gastrointest Endosc 2010; 71(6):983–9.

25. Sidhu R, Sanders DS. Double-balloon enteroscopy in the elderly with obscure gastrointestinal bleeding: safety and feasibility. Eur J Gastroenterol Hepatol 2013;25(10):1230–4.

26. Byeon JS, Mann NK, Jamil LH, et al. Double balloon enteroscopy can be safely done in elderly patients with significant co-morbidities. J Gastroenterol Hepatol 2012;27(12):1831–6.

27. Gurkan OE, Karakan T, Dogan I, et al. Comparison of double balloon enteroscopy in adults and children. World J Gastroenterol 2013;19(29):4726–31.

28. Sorser SA, Watson A, Gamarra RM, et al. Double balloon enteroscopy: is it efficacious and safe in a community setting? Minerva Gastroenterol Dietol 2013;59(2): 205–10.

29. Sanaka MR, Navaneethan U, Upchurch BR, et al. Diagnostic and therapeutic yield is not influenced by the timing of small-bowel enteroscopy: morning versus afternoon. Gastrointest Endosc 2013;77(1):62–70.

30. Rajan EA, Pais SA, Degregorio BT, et al. Small-bowel endoscopy core curriculum. Gastrointest Endosc 2013;77(1):1–6.

31. Anderson MA, Ben-Menachem T, Gan SI, et al. Management of antithrombotic agents for endoscopic procedures. Gastrointest Endosc 2009;70(6):1060–70.

32. Baron TH, Kamath PS, McBane RD. New anticoagulant and antiplatelet agents: a primer for the gastroenterologist. Clin Gastroenterol Hepatol 2014; 12(2):187–95.

33. Hirai F, Beppu T, Nishimura T, et al. Carbon dioxide insufflation compared with air insufflation in double-balloon enteroscopy: a prospective, randomized, double-blind trial. Gastrointest Endosc 2011;73(4):743–9.

34. Lenz P, Meister T, Manno M, et al. CO2 insufflation during single-balloon enteroscopy: a multicenter randomized controlled trial. Endoscopy 2014;46(1):53–8.

35. Tee HP, How SH, Kaffes AJ. Learning curve for double-balloon enteroscopy: findings from an analysis of 282 procedures. World J Gastrointest Endosc 2012;4(8): 368–72.

36. Gerson LB, Flodin JT, Miyabayashi K. Balloon-assisted enteroscopy: technology and troubleshooting. Gastrointest Endosc 2008;68(6):1158–67.

37. Mehdizadeh S, Ross A, Gerson L, et al. What is the learning curve associated with double-balloon enteroscopy? Technical details and early experience in 6 US tertiary care centers. Gastrointest Endosc 2006;64(5):740–50.

38. Manno M, Barbera C, Bertani H, et al. Single balloon enteroscopy: technical aspects and clinical applications. World J Gastrointest Endosc 2012;4(2):28–32.

39. Aktas H, Mensink PB. Therapeutic balloon-assisted enteroscopy. Dig Dis 2008; 26(4):309–13.

40. Akerman PA, Agrawal D, Chen W, et al. Spiral enteroscopy: a novel method of enteroscopy by using the Endo-Ease Discovery SB overtube and a pediatric colonoscope. Gastrointest Endosc 2009;69(2):327–32.

41. Mensink PB, Haringsma J, Kucharzik T, et al. Complications of double balloon enteroscopy: a multicenter survey. Endoscopy 2007;39(7):613–5.

42. Rondonotti E, Sunada K, Yano T, et al. Double-balloon endoscopy in clinical practice: where are we now? Dig Endosc 2012;24(4):209–19.

43. Nakayama S, Tominaga K, Obayashi T, et al. The prevalence of adverse events associated with double-balloon enteroscopy from a single-centre dataset in Japan. Dig Liver Dis 2014;46:706–9.

44. Onal IK, Akdogan M, Arhan M, et al. Double balloon enteroscopy: a 3-year experience at a tertiary care center. Hepatogastroenterology 2012;59(118):1851–4.

45. May A, Nachbar L, Pohl J, et al. Endoscopic interventions in the small bowel using double balloon enteroscopy: feasibility and limitations. Am J Gastroenterol 2007;102(3):527–35.

46. Aktas H, de Ridder L, Haringsma J, et al. Complications of single-balloon enteroscopy: a prospective evaluation of 166 procedures. Endoscopy 2010;42(5): 365–8.

47. Pohl J, Blancas JM, Cave D, et al. Consensus report of the 2nd International Conference on double balloon endoscopy. Endoscopy 2008;40(2):156–60.

48. Moschler O, May A, Muller MK, et al. Complications in and performance of double-balloon enteroscopy (DBE): results from a large prospective DBE database in Germany. Endoscopy 2011;43(6):484–9.

49. Gerson LB, Tokar J, Chiorean M, et al. Complications associated with double balloon enteroscopy at nine US centers. Clin Gastroenterol Hepatol 2009;7(11): 1177–82, 1182.e1–3.

50. Kopacova M, Tacheci I, Rejchrt S, et al. Double balloon enteroscopy and acute pancreatitis. World J Gastroenterol 2010;16(19):2331–40.

51. Itaba S, Nakamura K, Aso A, et al. Prospective, randomized, double-blind, placebo-controlled trial of ulinastatin for prevention of hyperenzymemia after double balloon endoscopy via the antegrade approach. Dig Endosc 2013;25(4):421–7.

52. Yip WM, Lok KH, Lai L, et al. Acute pancreatitis: rare complication of retrograde single-balloon enteroscopy. Endoscopy 2009;41(Suppl 2):E324.

53. Groenen MJ, Moreels TG, Orlent H, et al. Acute pancreatitis after double-balloon enteroscopy: an old pathogenetic theory revisited as a result of using a new endoscopic tool. Endoscopy 2006;38(1):82–5.

54. Teshima CW, Aktas H, Kuipers EJ, et al. Hyperamylasemia and pancreatitis following spiral enteroscopy. Can J Gastroenterol 2012;26(9):603–6.

55. Latorre R, Soria F, Lopez-Albors O, et al. Effect of double-balloon enteroscopy on pancreas: an experimental porcine model. World J Gastroenterol 2012;18(37): 5181–7.

56. Shibuya T, Osada T, Nomura O, et al. The origin of hyperamylasemia associated with peroral double-balloon endoscopy. J Clin Gastroenterol 2012;46(10):888–9.

57. Zepeda-Gomez S, Barreto-Zuniga R, Ponce-de-Leon S, et al. Risk of hyperamylasemia and acute pancreatitis after double-balloon enteroscopy: a prospective study. Endoscopy 2011;43(9):766–70.

58. Pata C, Akyuz U, Erzin Y, et al. Post-procedure elevated amylase and lipase levels after double-balloon enteroscopy: relations with the double-balloon technique. Dig Dis Sci 2010;55(7):1982–8.

59. Judah JR, Collins D, Gaidos JK, et al. Prospective evaluation of gastroenterologist-guided, nurse-administered standard sedation for spiral deep small bowel enteroscopy. Dig Dis Sci 2010;55(9):2584–91.

60. Yen HH, Chen YY, Su WW, et al. Intestinal necrosis as a complication of epinephrine injection therapy during double-balloon enteroscopy. Endoscopy 2006;38(5):542.

61. Hilzenrat N, Lamoureux E, Alpert L. Gastric ischemia after epinephrine injection for upper GI bleeding in a patient with unsuspected amyloidosis. Gastrointest Endosc 2003;58(2):307–8.

62. Arhan M, Akdogan M, Oguz D, et al. A rare complication of retrograde double-balloon enteroscopy: subcutaneous emphysema. Am J Gastroenterol 2008; 103(9):2409–10.

63. Izawa N, Kouro T, Sawada T, et al. Pneumobilia: a rare complication or a common phenomenon of double-balloon enteroscopy? Am J Gastroenterol 2009;104(8): 2122–3.

64. Chavalitdhamrong D, Draganov PV. Acute stroke due to air embolism complicating ERCP. Endoscopy 2013;45(Suppl 2 UCTN):E177–8.

65. Cheng DW, Han NJ, Mehdizadeh S, et al. Intraperitoneal bleeding after oral double-balloon enteroscopy: a case report and review of the literature. Gastrointest Endosc 2007;66(3):627–9.

66. Gondal B, Charpentier J, Cave D. Hematoperitoneum after small-bowel spiral enteroscopy. Endoscopy 2013;45(Suppl 2):E337.

67. Koksal AS, Kalkan IH, Torun S, et al. Superior mesenteric artery thrombosis related to double balloon enteroscopy in a patient with Crohn's disease. Clin Res Hepatol Gastroenterol 2013;37(1):e40–1.

68. Aktas H, Mensink PB, Haringsma J, et al. Low incidence of hyperamylasemia after proximal double-balloon enteroscopy: has the insertion technique improved? Endoscopy 2009;41(8):670–3.

69. Kopacova M, Rejchrt S, Tacheci I, et al. Hyperamylasemia of uncertain significance associated with oral double-balloon enteroscopy. Gastrointest Endosc 2007;66(6):1133–8.

70. Riccioni ME, Urgesi R, Cianci R, et al. Single-balloon push-and-pull enteroscopy system: does it work? A single-center, 3-year experience. Surg Endosc 2011; 25(9):3050–6.

71. Morgan D, Upchurch B, Draganov P, et al. Spiral enteroscopy: prospective US multicenter study in patients with small-bowel disorders. Gastrointest Endosc 2010;72(5):992–8.

72. Frieling T, Heise J, Sassenrath W, et al. Prospective comparison between double-balloon enteroscopy and spiral enteroscopy. Endoscopy 2010;42(11):885–8.

Endoscopic Retrograde Cholangiopancreatography– Related Adverse Events

General Overview

Tarun Rustagi, MD, Priya A. Jamidar, MD*

KEYWORDS

- ERCP • Risk factors • Sphincterotomy • Pancreatitis • Bleeding • Complications
- Cholangitiis • Perforation

KEY POINTS

- Diagnostic and therapeutic endoscopic retrograde cholangiopancreatography (ERCP) has been a major advance in medicine.
- A good understanding of patient-related and procedure-related risk factors is important for ERCP, as is the judicious selection of patients.
- Overall adverse event rates for ERCP are typically reported as 5–10%.
- The most commonly reported adverse events include post-ERCP pancreatitis, bleeding, perforation, cholangitis, and cardiopulomary or sedation related events.
- Strategies to minimize, recognize, and manage adverse events are key skills necessary for the practicing endoscopist.

INTRODUCTION

Endoscopic retrograde cholangiopancreatography (ERCP) was first performed in 1968 and the first sphincterotomy was carried out in 1974. ERCP has evolved into a routine endoscopic procedure, with approximately 500,000 procedures performed in the United States and 1.3 million worldwide annually. Most procedures in the United States are therapeutic. ERCP represents a monumental advance in the management of patients with pancreaticobiliary diseases, but is a complex and technically demanding procedure with the highest inherent risk for adverse events of all routine endoscopic procedures. This article evaluates patient-related and procedure-related

The authors disclose that there are no potential conflicts of interest (financial, professional, or personal) that are relevant to the article.

Section of Digestive Diseases, Department of Internal Medicine, Yale University School of Medicine, 333 Cedar Street, 1080 LMP, New Haven, CT 06520, USA

* Corresponding author. Section of Digestive Diseases, Yale University School of Medicine, 333 Cedar Street, 1080 LMP, PO Box 208019, New Haven, CT 06520-8019.

E-mail address: priya.jamidar@yale.edu

Gastrointest Endoscopy Clin N Am 25 (2015) 97–106

http://dx.doi.org/10.1016/j.giec.2014.09.005   **giendo.theclinics.com**

risk factors for ERCP-related adverse events, and discusses strategies for the diagnosis and management of these events.

GENERAL CONSIDERATIONS

Before considering performing an ERCP, the endoscopist must ensure there is an appropriate indication. There has been a dramatic reduction in diagnostic ERCPs given the increased use of less invasive imaging modalities to view the pancreaticobiliary system (eg, MRI, computed tomography, and endoscopic ultrasonography [EUS]). Endoscopists must also consider if they have adequate volume to maintain their ERCP skills and minimize adverse events. Overall adverse event rates for ERCP are typically reported as 5% to 10%. The most commonly reported complications include post-ERCP pancreatitis (PEP), bleeding, perforation, infection (cholangitis), and cardiopulmonary or sedation-related events. This article reviews these adverse events and its companion article elsewhere in this issue by Drs Rustagi and Jamidar focuses solely on PEP.

POST–ENDOSCOPIC RETROGRADE CHOLANGIOPANCREATOGRAPHY PANCREATITIS

Given the importance of this topic and the large amount of published data, PEP is covered in greater detail in the accompanying article by Drs Rustagi and Jamidar focuses on PEP. This section provides a brief overview of the subject.

PEP is one of the most common and feared adverse events of ERCP, resulting in considerable morbidity and, rarely, death. Several patient-related (younger age, female gender, history of previous PEP, nondilated ducts, normal bilirubin level, suspected sphincter of Oddi dysfunction) and procedure-related factors (difficult cannulation, multiple pancreatic injections, pancreatic sphincterotomy, precut sphincterotomy, pancreatic sampling) have been identified as increasing the risk of PEP.[1–9] Therefore, careful patient selection and sound endoscopic technique are the cornerstones in the prevention of PEP.

Prophylactic pancreatic duct stenting, particularly in high-risk patients, has been shown to reduce the incidence and severity of PEP by mechanically facilitating pancreatic drainage.[10–15]

In addition, chemoprophylaxis of PEP has been extensively researched in an attempt to prevent or reduce the severity of PEP. Numerous trials studying a variety of pharmacologic agents (eg, somatostatin, octreotide, corticosteroids, allopurinol, protease inhibitors, nitroglycerin) have yielded disappointing results[16–21]; however, an important exception is rectal administration of nonsteroidal anti-inflammatory drugs (NSAIDs), which have been shown in large randomized controlled trials and meta-analyses to significantly reduce the incidence and severity of PEP.[14,22–28]

BLEEDING

Bleeding observed at the time of or after ERCP is usually related to endoscopic sphincterotomy. Bleeding seen endoscopically during or immediately after sphincterotomy is not uncommon, but is generally not considered an adverse event unless there is clinically significant blood loss, transfusion, or a major change in management.

The true incidence of significant ERCP-related hemorrhage is variable and difficult to define given the lack of a standard definition. Some degree of bleeding (ranging from oozing to severe bleeding) is seen at the time of sphincterotomy in up to 10% to 30% of cases.[5] However, endoscopists are generally unconcerned about minor bleeding, such as limited oozing immediately after a sphincterotomy, because in most cases this is temporary and stops spontaneously.[4] When applying clinical criteria such as melena, hematemesis, a greater than 2 g/dL drop in hemoglobin level, or requirement for secondary intervention such as endoscopy or blood transfusion, the overall incidence of bleeding is around 0.1% to 2%.[3–5,7,8,29,30] Based on severity, bleeding has been classified into 4 groups: (1) mild (clinical evidence for bleeding but drop in hemoglobin is <3 g/dL; no blood transfusions), (2) moderate (endoscopic treatment required; transfusion requirement ≤4 units), (3) severe (transfusion of ≥5 units and/or surgery or angiographic treatment), and (4) fatal.[4,31]

Immediate bleeding, defined as continued bleeding 2 to 3 minutes after the initial sphincterotomy, is seen in 50% to 60% of patients.[5,30,32–35] Delayed bleeding, defined as occurring after the completion of ERCP, can happen hours or up to 7 to 10 days after the procedure.[5,30,32,35]

Several risks for postsphincterotomy hemorrhage have been identified, which allow risk-stratification and risk-reduction measures to be taken before the procedure. Definite risk factors include any degree of bleeding during the procedure, presence of any coagulopathy or thrombocytopenia, initiation of anticoagulant therapy within 3 days after the sphincterotomy, presence of active cholangitis, and endoscopist's low case volume (performance of <1 sphincterotomy per week).[5,30] Other potential risk factors include ampullary stone impaction, periampullary diverticula, uncontrolled cutting (the so-called zipper cut), and needle-knife sphincterotomy.[2,4,36,37] Factors that do not seem to increase risk of bleeding include longer sphincterotomy incision, extension of a previous sphincterotomy, and use of aspirin or NSAIDs.[5,30] The risk of bleeding with newer agents including clopidogrel is unclear.

In patients with thrombocytopenia or coagulopathy, risk can be minimized by transfusion of blood products (with goal of platelet counts >50,000/mm^3 and international normalized ratio <1.5–2), withholding anticoagulants for 3 days afterward, and avoiding sphincterotomy by use of alternative procedures such as balloon sphincteroplasty.[4,5] Prophylactic epinephrine injection into the sphincterotomy site in high-risk patients has been suggested to reduce the risk of postsphincterotomy bleeding but is of uncertain efficacy.[5] Intraprocedurally, the use of blended current through automated current delivery cautery systems has been shown to reduce the risk of immediate bleeding.[5,32,35]

Many types of endoscopic therapies are available for immediate or delayed postsphincterotomy hemorrhage. Injection of dilute epinephrine (1:10,000) is the most common first-line endoscopic approach.[5,34,35] Varying amounts are injected at a targeted site or in the apex of the sphincterotomy site if bleeding obscures visualization. Needles with a metal shaft and spring sheath (Carr-Locke injection needle; US Endoscopy, Mentor, OH, USA) may pass more easily through the tip and elevator of the side-viewing duodenoscope. A comparison between epinephrine injection monotherapy and combination endotherapy (epinephrine plus cautery) was retrospectively evaluated in a single-center experience, resulting in similar rates of success (96.2% vs 100%; $P = .44$), recurrent hemorrhage (16% vs 12.1%; $P = .72$), other procedural adverse events, transfusions, angiographic embolization, and surgery.[38]

Balloon tamponade using a standard stone extraction or dilation balloon may allow control of bleeding and improve visualization of the bleeding site. Thermal coaptive coagulation using either a multipolar probe or heater probe device can follow, particularly if a specific bleeding point can be identified. Endoscopic clip placement is another option, and can be very effective. Caution should be taken to avoid thermal injury or clip placement over the pancreatic duct orifice, especially if the bleeding site is to the right of the sphincterotomy incision contiguous to the pancreatic duct orifice. Fully covered self-expandable metallic stents (FCSEMS) have also been used with success to create a tamponade effect at the area of bleeding as a rescue technique if other endoscopic methods have failed.[39–41] Application of a catheter-delivered hemostatic powder, TC-325 (Hemospray; Cook Medical, Winston-Salem, NC, USA), is a promising potential therapy for hemostasis of sphincterotomy-induced hemorrhage but is not currently available in the United States.[42,43] Rarely, angiographic embolization or surgery is required for refractory bleeding.

PERFORATION

Perforation is an uncommon adverse event, occurring in 0.3% to 0.6% of cases.[4,7,8,44,45] Three distinct types of perforations can occur: (1) free wall perforation of the esophagus, stomach, or duodenum by the endoscope, resulting in mediastinal or intraperitoneal leakage; (2) retroperitoneal perforation as a result of extension of a sphincterotomy incision beyond the intramural portion of the bile or pancreatic duct; and (3) perforation of the bile or pancreatic duct from extramural passage of guide wires or stents.

Bowel wall perforations are force and angle related, and are more likely to occur in patients with esophageal stricture, Zenker diverticulum, postsurgical altered anatomy with fixed angulation, or gastric outlet obstruction caused by advanced pancreatic cancer.[4,35,46] The duodenum is the most common site of free bowel wall perforation, which typically occurs with mechanical pressure from a rigid duodenoscope tip tearing a thin-walled proximal duodenum, or when the scope tip tears a periampullary diverticulum. Sphincterotomy-related perforations are more common after needle-knife precut access, and in patients with suspected sphincter of Oddi dysfunction.[5,47] Guide wire–related ductal perforations typically occur through a side branch of the pancreatic duct or hepatic capsule, but have become less common with increasing use of floppy-tipped, hydrophilic wires. Dilation of biliary or pancreatic duct strictures and the use of a large extraction balloon in a small-caliber duct can also lead to intraductal rupture.

Treatment of post-ERCP perforation depends on the type, size, and location of the perforation and severity of the leak, clinical manifestations and stability of the patient, and available devices and expertise. This topic is also covered in the article discussing perforation closure and management elsewhere in this issue. Early recognition and endoscopic treatment of suspected perforation along with conservative management has been shown to have favorable outcomes.[45,47] Although free bowel wall perforations have been managed historically with surgical repair, improved endoscopic closure devices have permitted nonsurgical management in an increasing number of cases, particularly if the perforation is recognized at the time of the endoscopy.

Attempts to close perforations endoscopically should be performed using CO_2 to minimize the risk of tension pneumoperitoneum or extensive retroperitoneal, mediastinal, and subcutaneous gas accumulation, including pneumothorax. Several reports supporting the primary endoscopic closure techniques using an endoscopic clip, endoloop, or the over-the-scope clip (OTSC) to treat larger perforations have been described, even for use in direct perforation of the duodenal wall.[48,49] The OTSC (Ovesco Endoscopy AG, Tübingen, Germany; Padlock, Aponos Medical, Kingston NH, USA), have been successfully used for closure of esophageal, gastric, and duodenal perforations.[50–52] The OTSC enables more durable closure than the through-the-scope clip because of its ability to grasp more tissue (by pulling the defect edges into the cap before clip deployment) and apply a greater compression force for closure.[52,53] Endoscopic suturing (OverStitch; Apollo Endosurgery, Austin, TX, USA) is an option for accurate endoscopic full-thickness closure of iatrogenic perforations, though suturing is limited by the availability of the device, length of the dual-channel upper endoscope, and difficulty in operating within the narrow duodenal lumen.[54] In addition, FCSEMS have also been used successfully to close esophageal and, more specifically, scope-induced duodenal wall perforations.[35,41,55]

Wire-related ductal perforations can usually be treated endoscopically by inserting a stent in the respective duct and providing transduodenal duct drainage beyond the leak site.[5,45,47] Sphincterotomy-related perforation may be minimized by limiting the length of cutting wire in contact with the tissue, using stepwise incisions, and using the newer-generation microprocessor-controlled electrosurgical generators.[5,35] The safety profiles of cutting currents provided by these generators have eliminated any need to use a pure cut setting. If perforation is suspected during a sphincterotomy, careful fluoroscopy and injection of a small amount of contrast while pulling the papillotome through the incision over a guide wire can confirm or exclude extravasation. Endoscopic clipping may be attempted to close a definite leak.[5,47] An FCSEMS can also be placed to drain the bile duct and occlude the leak site in biliary sphincterotomy-related perforation.[41,47,55]

In addition to endotherapy, patients should be admitted, kept nil by mouth with nasogastric suction, given intravenous acid-suppressive therapy and intravenous antibiotics, and have a surgical consultation. Furthermore, abdominal computed tomography should be obtained to assess for the degree of contrast leakage, fluid collection, and inflammation. If there is significant leak with ongoing contrast extravasation, or deterioration in a patient's clinical condition, prompt surgical or percutaneous drainage is recommended.

INFECTIONS

Infectious complications of ERCP include acute cholangitis and cholecystitis, with a reported incidence of less than 2% in larger case series.[4,7,8,44] The most important risk factor for post-ERCP acute cholangitis is failed or incomplete biliary drainage.[3,5,7,8,30,35,56] Additional risk factors for ERCP-related biliary infections include jaundice, especially if caused by malignancy; primary sclerosing cholangitis (because of poor drainage of injected contrast from a strictured biliary tree); endoscopist inexperience; and the performance of a rendezvous (combined percutaneous/endoscopic) procedure.[4,30] Routine antibiotic prophylaxis provides no clinical benefit in patients with successful drainage and without antecedent cholangitis; however, broad-spectrum antibiotics with gram-negative coverage should be administered in all cases with incomplete biliary drainage.[57–59]

The risk of post-ERCP biliary infections can be reduced by: (1) aspirating and lavaging infected bile from an obstructed system before contrast injection to avoid an increase in intraductal pressure, which can lead to translocation of biliary bacteria into the bloodstream; (2) minimizing the volume of contrast injected into the biliary tree; and (3) achieving prompt endoscopic decompression of an obstructed biliary system and, if complete biliary drainage is not feasible, undertaking percutaneous or surgical intervention without delay.[4]

Cholecystitis is less frequently reported than acute cholangitis after ERCP. Placement of an FCSEMS has been associated with cholecystitis; however, this is more likely related to tumor involvement of the cystic duct orifice, regardless of the type of stent.[60–62] Once recognized, cholecystitis can be managed conservatively, surgically, by percutaneous drainage, or endoscopically (EUS-guided endoluminal drainage or transpapillary gallbladder drainage at ERCP).[61,63]

OTHER ADVERSE EVENTS

Cardiopulmonary Events

Cardiopulmonary events are a leading cause of deaths related to ERCP, but are often underemphasized and overlooked by endoscopists. These events are often associated with sedation, and occur in as many as 0.9% to 1.33% of all ERCPs.[44,64] This frequency is greater relative to general endoscopy procedures, given the requirement of deeper sedation over a longer period of time, often in elderly patients with multiple comorbidities. Higher risk of aspiration from concomitant gastric outlet obstruction in patients with advanced pancreatobiliary malignancies might also contribute to a higher rate of cardiopulmonary complications.

Increasingly, propofol and anesthesiologist-administered sedation is being used for ERCP. Several studies comparing different types of anesthesia have yielded conflicting results. Research has included examining different combinations for conscious sedation, conscious sedation or propofol sedation, and nurse-administered or gastroenterologist-administered anesthesia.[65–68] In general, appropriate risk assessment should be performed in all patients to minimize the cardiopulmonary and sedation-related adverse events, and endotracheal intubation with general anesthesia should be used when indicated.

Miscellaneous Events

A large number of rare adverse events complicating ERCP have been described, including: systemic air and bile embolism; contrast allergy; cannulation and opacification of the portal vein and hepatic artery; hepatic and splenic trauma; gallstone ileus; and intestinal pneumatosis, pneumothorax, pneumomediastinum, and pneumoperitoneum.[4,53]

SUMMARY

Diagnostic and therapeutic ERCP has been a major advance in medicine. A good understanding of patient-related and procedure-related risk factors is important, as is the judicious selection of patients for ERCP. Strategies to minimize, recognize, and manage adverse events are key skills necessary for the practicing endoscopist.

REFERENCES

1. Freeman ML, DiSario JA, Nelson DB, et al. Risk factors for post-ERCP pancreatitis: a prospective, multicenter study. Gastrointest Endosc 2001;54:425–34.
2. Masci E, Toti G, Mariani A, et al. Complications of diagnostic and therapeutic ERCP: a prospective multicenter study. Am J Gastroenterol 2001;96:417–23.
3. Loperfido S, Angelini G, Benedetti G, et al. Major early complications from diagnostic and therapeutic ERCP: a prospective multicenter study. Gastrointest Endosc 1998;48:1–10.
4. Mergener K. Complications of endoscopic and radiologic investigation of biliary tract disorders. Curr Gastroenterol Rep 2011;13:173–81.
5. Freeman ML. Complications of endoscopic retrograde cholangiopancreatography: avoidance and management. Gastrointest Endosc Clin N Am 2012;22: 567–86.
6. Cheng CL, Sherman S, Watkins JL, et al. Risk factors for post-ERCP pancreatitis: a prospective multicenter study. Am J Gastroenterol 2006;101:139–47.
7. Wang P, Li ZS, Liu F, et al. Risk factors for ERCP-related complications: a prospective multicenter study. Am J Gastroenterol 2009;104:31–40.

8. Williams EJ, Taylor S, Fairclough P, et al. Risk factors for complication following ERCP; results of a large-scale, prospective multicenter study. Endoscopy 2007; 39:793–801.

9. Masci E, Mariani A, Curioni S, et al. Risk factors for pancreatitis following endoscopic retrograde cholangiopancreatography: a meta-analysis. Endoscopy 2003;35:830–4.

10. Bhatia V, Ahuja V, Acharya SK, et al. A randomized controlled trial of valdecoxib and glyceryl trinitrate for the prevention of post-ERCP pancreatitis. J Clin Gastroenterol 2011;45:170–6.

11. Fazel A, Quadri A, Catalano MF, et al. Does a pancreatic duct stent prevent post-ERCP pancreatitis? A prospective randomized study. Gastrointest Endosc 2003;57:291–4.

12. Singh P, Das A, Isenberg G, et al. Does prophylactic pancreatic stent placement reduce the risk of post-ERCP acute pancreatitis? A meta-analysis of controlled trials. Gastrointest Endosc 2004;60:544–50.

13. Tarnasky PR. Mechanical prevention of post-ERCP pancreatitis by pancreatic stents: results, techniques, and indications. JOP 2003;4:58–67.

14. Akbar A, Abu Dayyeh BK, Baron TH, et al. Rectal nonsteroidal anti-inflammatory drugs are superior to pancreatic duct stents in preventing pancreatitis after endoscopic retrograde cholangiopancreatography: a network meta-analysis. Clin Gastroenterol Hepatol 2013;11:778–83.

15. Choudhary A, Bechtold ML, Arif M, et al. Pancreatic stents for prophylaxis against post-ERCP pancreatitis: a meta-analysis and systematic review. Gastrointest Endosc 2011;73:275–82.

16. Sternlieb JM, Aronchick CA, Retig JN, et al. A multicenter, randomized, controlled trial to evaluate the effect of prophylactic octreotide on ERCP-induced pancreatitis. Am J Gastroenterol 1992;87:1561–6.

17. Andriulli A, Leandro G, Federici T, et al. Prophylactic administration of somatostatin or gabexate does not prevent pancreatitis after ERCP: an updated meta-analysis. Gastrointest Endosc 2007;65:624–32.

18. Sherman S, Blaut U, Watkins JL, et al. Does prophylactic administration of corticosteroid reduce the risk and severity of post-ERCP pancreatitis: a randomized, prospective, multicenter study. Gastrointest Endosc 2003;58:23–9.

19. Shao LM, Chen QY, Chen MY, et al. Nitroglycerin in the prevention of post-ERCP pancreatitis: a meta-analysis. Dig Dis Sci 2010;55:1–7.

20. Yuhara H, Ogawa M, Kawaguchi Y, et al. Pharmacologic prophylaxis of post-endoscopic retrograde cholangiopancreatography pancreatitis: protease inhibitors and NSAIDs in a meta-analysis. J Gastroenterol 2014;49:388–99.

21. Omata F, Deshpande G, Tokuda Y, et al. Meta-analysis: somatostatin or its long-acting analogue, octreotide, for prophylaxis against post-ERCP pancreatitis. J Gastroenterol 2010;45:885–95.

22. Ahmad D, Lopez KT, Esmadi MA, et al. The effect of indomethacin in the prevention of post-endoscopic retrograde cholangiopancreatography pancreatitis: a meta-analysis. Pancreas 2014;43:338–42.

23. Elmunzer BJ, Scheiman JM, Lehman GA, et al. A randomized trial of rectal indomethacin to prevent post-ERCP pancreatitis. N Engl J Med 2012;366:1414–22.

24. Puig I, Calvet X, Baylina M, et al. How and when should NSAIDs be used for preventing post-ERCP pancreatitis? A systematic review and meta-analysis. PLoS One 2014;9:e92922.

25. Sethi S, Sethi N, Wadhwa V, et al. A meta-analysis on the role of rectal diclofenac and indomethacin in the prevention of post-endoscopic retrograde cholangiopancreatography pancreatitis. Pancreas 2014;43:190–7.

26. Sotoudehmanesh R, Khatibian M, Kolahdoozan S, et al. Indomethacin may reduce the incidence and severity of acute pancreatitis after ERCP. Am J Gastroenterol 2007;102:978–83.

27. Yaghoobi M, Rolland S, Waschke KA, et al. Meta-analysis: rectal indomethacin for the prevention of post-ERCP pancreatitis. Aliment Pharmacol Ther 2013;38: 995–1001.

28. Ding X, Chen M, Huang S, et al. Nonsteroidal anti-inflammatory drugs for prevention of post-ERCP pancreatitis: a meta-analysis. Gastrointest Endosc 2012;76: 1152–9.

29. Christensen M, Matzen P, Schulze S, et al. Complications of ERCP: a prospective study. Gastrointest Endosc 2004;60:721–31.

30. Freeman ML, Nelson DB, Sherman S, et al. Complications of endoscopic biliary sphincterotomy. N Engl J Med 1996;335:909–18.

31. Cotton PB, Lehman G, Vennes J, et al. Endoscopic sphincterotomy complications and their management: an attempt at consensus. Gastrointest Endosc 1991;37: 383–93.

32. Freeman ML. Adverse outcomes of ERCP. Gastrointest Endosc 2002;56: S273–82.

33. Ferreira LE, Fatima J, Baron TH. Clinically significant delayed postsphincterotomy bleeding: a twelve year single center experience. Minerva Gastroenterol Dietol 2007;53:215–23.

34. Vasconez C, Llach J, Bordas JM, et al. Injection treatment of hemorrhage induced by endoscopic sphincterotomy. Endoscopy 1998;30:37–9.

35. Balmadrid B, Kozarek R. Prevention and management of adverse events of endoscopic retrograde cholangiopancreatography. Gastrointest Endosc Clin N Am 2013;23:385–403.

36. Kim HJ, Kim MH, Kim DI, et al. Endoscopic hemostasis in sphincterotomy-induced hemorrhage: its efficacy and safety. Endoscopy 1999;31:431–6.

37. Katsinelos P, Kountouras J, Chatzimavroudis G, et al. A novel technique of injection treatment for endoscopic sphincterotomy-induced hemorrhage. Endoscopy 2007;39:631–6.

38. Tsou YK, Lin CH, Liu NJ, et al. Treating delayed endoscopic sphincterotomy-induced bleeding: epinephrine injection with or without thermotherapy. World J Gastroenterol 2009;15:4823–8.

39. Itoi T, Yasuda I, Doi S, et al. Endoscopic hemostasis using covered metallic stent placement for uncontrolled post-endoscopic sphincterotomy bleeding. Endoscopy 2011;43:369–72.

40. Shah JN, Marson F, Binmoeller KF. Temporary self-expandable metal stent placement for treatment of post-sphincterotomy bleeding. Gastrointest Endosc 2010; 72:1274–8.

41. Canena J, Liberato M, Horta D, et al. Short-term stenting using fully covered self-expandable metal stents for treatment of refractory biliary leaks, postsphincterotomy bleeding, and perforations. Surg Endosc 2013;27:313–24.

42. Appleby VJ, Hutchinson JM, Beckett CJ, et al. Use of the haemostatic agent TC-325 in the treatment of bleeding secondary to endoscopic retrograde cholangiopancreatography sphincterotomy. QJM 2014. [Epub ahead of print].

43. Moosavi S, Chen YI, Barkun AN. TC-325 application leading to transient obstruction of a post-sphincterotomy biliary orifice. Endoscopy 2013;45(Suppl 2 UCTN):E130.

44. Andriulli A, Loperfido S, Napolitano G, et al. Incidence rates of post-ERCP complications: a systematic survey of prospective studies. Am J Gastroenterol 2007; 102:1781–8.

45. Enns R, Eloubeidi MA, Mergener K, et al. ERCP-related perforations: risk factors and management. Endoscopy 2002;34:293–8.
46. Faylona JM, Qadir A, Chan AC, et al. Small-bowel perforations related to endoscopic retrograde cholangiopancreatography (ERCP) in patients with Billroth II gastrectomy. Endoscopy 1999;31:546–9.
47. Howard TJ, Tan T, Lehman GA, et al. Classification and management of perforations complicating endoscopic sphincterotomy. Surgery 1999;126:658–63 [discussion: 664–5].
48. Lee TH, Han JH, Park SH. Endoscopic treatments of endoscopic retrograde cholangiopancreatography-related duodenal perforations. Clin Endosc 2013; 46:522–8.
49. Mangiavillano B, Viaggi P, Masci E. Endoscopic closure of acute iatrogenic perforations during diagnostic and therapeutic endoscopy in the gastrointestinal tract using metallic clips: a literature review. J Dig Dis 2010;11:12–8.
50. Hagel AF, Naegel A, Lindner AS, et al. Over-the-scope clip application yields a high rate of closure in gastrointestinal perforations and may reduce emergency surgery. J Gastrointest Surg 2012;16:2132–8.
51. Gubler C, Bauerfeind P. Endoscopic closure of iatrogenic gastrointestinal tract perforations with the over-the-scope clip. Digestion 2012;85:302–7.
52. Weiland T, Fehlker M, Gottwald T, et al. Performance of the OTSC System in the endoscopic closure of iatrogenic gastrointestinal perforations: a systematic review. Surg Endosc 2013;27:2258–74.
53. Chavalitdhamrong D, Donepudi S, Pu L, et al. Uncommon and rarely reported adverse events of endoscopic retrograde cholangiopancreatography. Dig Endosc 2014;26:15–22.
54. Kumar N, Thompson CC. A novel method for endoscopic perforation management by using abdominal exploration and full-thickness sutured closure. Gastrointest Endosc 2014;80:156–61.
55. Vezakis A, Fragulidis G, Nastos C, et al. Closure of a persistent sphincterotomy-related duodenal perforation by placement of a covered self-expandable metallic biliary stent. World J Gastroenterol 2011;17:4539–41.
56. Boender J, Nix GA, de Ridder MA, et al. Endoscopic sphincterotomy and biliary drainage in patients with cholangitis due to common bile duct stones. Am J Gastroenterol 1995;90:233–8.
57. Bai Y, Gao F, Gao J, et al. Prophylactic antibiotics cannot prevent endoscopic retrograde cholangiopancreatography-induced cholangitis: a meta-analysis. Pancreas 2009;38:126–30.
58. ASGE Standards of Practice Committee, Banerjee S, Shen B, et al. Antibiotic prophylaxis for GI endoscopy. Gastrointest Endosc 2008;67:791–8.
59. Brand M, Bizos D, O'Farrell P Jr. Antibiotic prophylaxis for patients undergoing elective endoscopic retrograde cholangiopancreatography. Cochrane Database Syst Rev 2010;(10):CD007345.
60. Isayama H, Komatsu Y, Tsujino T, et al. A prospective randomised study of "covered" versus "uncovered" diamond stents for the management of distal malignant biliary obstruction. Gut 2004;53:729–34.
61. Saxena P, Singh VK, Lennon AM, et al. Endoscopic management of acute cholecystitis after metal stent placement in patients with malignant biliary obstruction: a case series. Gastrointest Endosc 2013;78:175–8.
62. Isayama H, Kawabe T, Nakai Y, et al. Cholecystitis after metallic stent placement in patients with malignant distal biliary obstruction. Clin Gastroenterol Hepatol 2006;4:1148–53.

63. Widmer J, Singhal S, Gaidhane M, et al. Endoscopic ultrasound-guided endoluminal drainage of the gallbladder. Dig Endosc 2014;26(4):525–31.
64. Kapral C, Duller C, Wewalka F, et al. Case volume and outcome of endoscopic retrograde cholangiopancreatography: results of a nationwide Austrian benchmarking project. Endoscopy 2008;40:625–30.
65. Sorser SA, Fan DS, Tommolino EE, et al. Complications of ERCP in patients undergoing general anesthesia versus MAC. Dig Dis Sci 2014;59:696–7.
66. Sethi S, Wadhwa V, Thaker A, et al. Propofol versus traditional sedative agents for advanced endoscopic procedures: a meta-analysis. Dig Endosc 2013; 26(4):515–24.
67. Guimaraes ES, Campbell EJ, Richter JM. The safety of nurse-administered procedural sedation compared to anesthesia care in a historical cohort of advanced endoscopy patients. Anesth Analg 2014;119(2):349–56.
68. Garewal D, Powell S, Milan SJ, et al. Sedative techniques for endoscopic retrograde cholangiopancreatography. Cochrane Database Syst Rev 2012;(6):CD007274.

Endoscopic Retrograde Cholangiopancreatography (ERCP)-Related Adverse Events
Post-ERCP Pancreatitis

Tarun Rustagi, MD, Priya A. Jamidar, MD*

KEYWORDS

- Pancreatitis • Indomethacin • Pancreatic stents • Sphincterotomy • Manometry
- Precut • Cannulation • Sphincter of Oddi dysfunction

KEY POINTS

- Post–endoscopic retrograde cholangiopancreatography pancreatitis (PEP), the most common complication of endoscopic retrograde cholangiopancreatography (ERCP), can be extremely serious, and may lead to long-term morbidity and even death.
- Diagnostic ERCP should be generally avoided, with few exceptions such as when accompanied by sphincter of Oddi manometry.
- Careful and judicious patient selection is paramount.
- The endoscopist must exercise meticulous technique, and patients deemed to be at high risk for PEP should receive rectal indomethacin and pancreatic stenting.
- Early recognition of PEP should initiate prompt supportive treatment.

INTRODUCTION

Post–endoscopic retrograde cholangiopancreatography pancreatitis (PEP) is one of the most common and feared adverse events related to endoscopic retrograde cholangiopancreatography (ERCP), resulting in considerable morbidity and, rarely, death. The reported rate of PEP varies widely from 1% to 40%, with an average rate of 5% to 7% seen in most observational and retrospective studies.[1–11] In a recent systematic review of 108 randomized controlled trials, which included 13,296 patients undergoing

Conflicts of Interest/Financial Disclosures/Funding/Grant Support/Writing Assistance: None. The authors disclose that there are no potential conflicts (financial, professional, or personal) that are relevant to the article.
Section of Digestive Diseases, Department of Internal Medicine, Yale University School of Medicine, 333 Cedar Street, 1080 LMP, New Haven, CT 06520, USA
* Corresponding author. Section of Digestive Diseases, Yale University School of Medicine, 333 Cedar Street, 1080 LMP, PO Box 208019, New Haven, CT 06520-8019.
E-mail address: priya.jamidar@yale.edu

Gastrointest Endoscopy Clin N Am 25 (2015) 107–121
http://dx.doi.org/10.1016/j.giec.2014.09.006
giendo.theclinics.com

both diagnostic and therapeutic ERCP, the overall rate of PEP was found to be 9.7%, with a mortality rate of 0.7% in the control group (placebo or no-pancreatic duct stent arms).[12] PEP remains a serious health problem, accounting for health care expenditures in excess of $150 million annually in the United States.[13]

Physicians and patients alike should be aware that not all pain following ERCP is PEP. Similarly, transient hyperamylasemia without acute pancreatitis is common after ERCP. PEP is defined as new or increased abdominal pain that is clinically consistent with acute pancreatitis (typically epigastric pain radiating to the to the back), associated with a serum amylase at least 3 times normal at more than 24 hours after the ERCP, and requiring hospital admission or prolongation of a planned admission.[2,8] The majority (80%–85%) of PEP cases are "mild" (requiring only up to 3 days of hospitalization). The remainder of PEP cases are described as either "moderately severe" (requiring 4–10 days' hospitalization) or "severe" (requiring >10 days' hospitalization), and these are associated with local and systemic complications.[8]

MECHANISMS OF POST–ENDOSCOPIC RETROGRADE CHOLANGIOPANCREATOGRAPHY PANCREATITIS

Several mechanisms of injury to the pancreas during ERCP have been postulated in the pathogenesis of PEP. A "trigger event" sets off a cascade of inflammatory activation similarly to acute pancreatitis from other causes. The initial triggering event could result from a variety of mechanisms listed in **Box 1**.

RISK FACTORS FOR POST–ENDOSCOPIC RETROGRADE CHOLANGIOPANCREATOGRAPHY PANCREATITIS

Large observational studies and randomized controlled trials have contributed to our understanding of the pathogenesis of PEP, with identification of several risk factors that are independently associated with the development of PEP. PEP depends on patient-related and procedure-related factors and the type of interventions done, and is perhaps also operator-dependent. **Box 2** summarizes the risk factors for PEP. Identification of preprocedure and intraprocedure risk factors allows risk stratification of patients and implementation of appropriate measures to reduce the incidence and severity of PEP, particularly in high-risk groups.

Patient-Related Factors

The patient-specific risk factors that have been associated with higher rates of PEP on multivariate analyses include younger age (<60 years), female gender, history of

---

Box 1
Postulated mechanisms of PEP

- Mechanical obstruction to the outflow of pancreatic secretions secondary to trauma, edema, or spasm of pancreatic sphincter
- Thermal injury from electrocautery during sphincterotomy
- Increased hydrostatic pressure in pancreatic duct from contrast injection or manometry without aspiration
- Ductal trauma and disruption from guide-wire manipulation
- Infection from introduction of duodenal flora into the pancreatic duct
- Chemical injury from contrast

Box 2
Risk factors for post-ERCP pancreatitis

Patient-Related Factors

- Younger age
- Female gender
- Suspected sphincter of Oddi dysfunction
- Normal serum bilirubin
- Prior post-ERCP pancreatitis
- History of recurrent acute pancreatitis
- Absence of chronic pancreatitis

Procedure-Related Factors

- Difficult cannulation
- Precut (access) sphincterotomy
- Pancreatic sphincterotomy
- Pancreatic guide-wire placement
- Pancreatic tissue sampling
- Multiple pancreatic injections
- Balloon dilation of intact biliary sphincter
- Endoscopic papillectomy/ampullectomy

---

previous PEP, nondilated ducts, normal bilirubin level, and suspected sphincter of Oddi dysfunction (SOD).[2–7,9,10,13,14] On the other hand, chronic pancreatitis, particularly chronic calcific pancreatitis and pancreatic malignancy, seem to be protective against PEP, likely because of decreased exocrine enzymatic activity and atrophy of the upstream pancreatic parenchyma from chronic obstruction.[4,15] Presence of pancreas divisum (unless dorsal duct cannulation is attempted), periampullary diverticulum, Billroth II gastrectomy, allergy to contrast media, and biliary interventions in patients with a preexisting biliary sphincterotomy are not associated with an increased risk of PEP.[5,16]

Patients with suspected SOD, particularly women, not only carry the highest risk for PEP, ranging from 10% to 40%, but are also more likely to develop severe pancreatitis and death.[2] In the landmark study by Freeman and colleagues[5] that included 2347 patients, PEP occurred in 52 of 272 (19.1%) patients with suspected SOD, and was found to be the most powerful risk factor for PEP (odds ratio [OR] 5.01, 95% confidence interval [CI] 2.73–9.22) on multivariate analysis. Although the exact reasons for such high risk remain unclear, the risk is similar with diagnostic, manometric, or therapeutic ERCP in these patients.

The risk of PEP appears to be higher among women, but this finding is confounded by the presence of SOD, which occurs much more frequently in women. In the aforementioned study by Freeman and colleagues,[5] female gender was significant on univariate analysis but not on multivariate analysis. However, a subsequent prospective, multicenter study by Freeman and colleagues,[4] including 1963 ERCP procedures, found female gender to be a significant risk factor on both univariate and multivariate analyses (OR 2.51, 95% CI 1.49–4.24; $P = .0001$). Female gender was also shown to be a significant risk factor for PEP (relative risk [RR] 2.23, 95% CI 1.75–2.84; P<.001) along with suspected SOD (RR 4.09, 95% CI 3.37–4.96) and previous pancreatitis (RR 2.46, 95% CI 1.93–3.12) in a meta-analysis of 15 prospective clinical studies with more than 10,000 patients.[7]

Procedure-Related Factors

Difficult cannulation, multiple pancreatic injections, pancreatic duct instrumentation, pancreatic sphincterotomy including minor papilla sphincterotomy, pancreatic sampling, and balloon dilation of an intact biliary sphincter have been identified as procedure-related factors that independently increase the risks of PEP.[2–7,10,14,17,18]

Papillary trauma induced by multiple attempts at cannulation appears to be a risk factor independent of the number of contrast injections into the pancreatic duct. In a large, prospective, multicenter study including 2347 patients, Freeman and colleagues[5] found difficultly in cannulation to be a significant risk factor for PEP (adjusted OR 2.40, 95% CI 1.07–5.36). The rates of PEP were higher with difficult (>15 attempts) or moderately difficult cannulation (6–15 attempts) in comparison with easy cannulation (≤5 attempts). The rates of PEP were 13%, 7%, and 3%, respectively.[5] In addition, the extent of pancreatic ductal opacification has been shown to correlate with the frequency of PEP. A retrospective analysis of 14,331 ERCPs showed that patients with opacification of head only (n = 845) had significantly lower incidence of PEP (3.6% vs 8.6%; P<.001) compared with those who had opacification to the tail of the pancreas (n = 4686).[19] However, acinarization of the pancreas may be less important than previously thought, and has not been found to be significant in large studies.[2,5,14]

Balloon dilation of an intact biliary sphincter has been associated with a markedly increased risk of PEP.[18,20,21] In one large randomized, controlled multicenter study of 117 patients assigned to dilation and 120 to sphincterotomy, there was a significantly increased rate of PEP in the balloon dilation group when compared with the sphincterotomy group (15.4% vs 0.8%), along with 2 deaths (1.7%) from pancreatitis following dilation, leading to termination of the study at the first interim analysis.[18] A subsequent Cochrane systematic review including 15 randomized trials (1768 participants) confirmed a higher risk of PEP, associated with endoscopic balloon dilation, in comparison with endoscopic sphincterotomy (RR 1.96, 95% CI 1.34–2.89).[22] However, balloon dilation after biliary sphincterotomy does not appear to increase the risk of PEP, and therefore is the preferred approach for extraction of large stones, particularly in patients with coagulopathy.[23–25]

Although patients with SOD have higher rates of PEP, contrary to widely held opinion, sphincter of Oddi manometry in itself does not carry a significant additional risk. With the widespread use of aspiration instead of conventional perfusion manometry catheters, the risk of hydrostatic injury and PEP with biliary and pancreatic sphincter manometry has probably been reduced to that of cannulation with any other ERCP accessory.[5] In an early randomized trial including 76 patients, sphincter of Oddi manometry using the aspiration catheter was associated with a significantly decreased frequency of PEP (23.5% vs 3%, P = .01), reduced mean hospital stay (5 ± 1.83 days; P = .03), and milder pancreatitis, compared with the standard perfusion system.[26] Studies comparing the risk of PEP in patients having ERCP for suspected SOD with and without sphincter of Oddi manometry have shown no independent risk of manometry in addition to the high risk conferred from underlying SOD itself. In a large retrospective analysis of 11,497 ERCPs performed over 12 years, neither pancreatic (OR 1.43, 95% CI 0.99–2.08) nor biliary manometry (1.16, 95% CI 0.83–1.62) was found to be a statistically significant risk factor for PEP.[9]

Data regarding the risk of PEP associated with the use of biliary self-expanding metal stents (SEMS) is conflicting, with rates ranging from 0% to 9%.[27–31] Theoretically the large diameter and radial expansion of the SEMS can obstruct or distort the pancreatic orifice or common channel, leading to PEP. In a retrospective study of 544 patients with malignant biliary obstruction, the frequency of PEP was significantly higher in the SEMS group than in the plastic stent group (7.3% vs 1.3%, respectively; OR 5.7, 95% CI 1.9–17.1).[27] The frequency of PEP was similar between covered (6.9%) and uncovered (7.5%) SEMS (OR 0.9, 95% CI 0.3–2.4).[27] In another retrospective study, pancreatitis following SEMS insertion was observed in 22 of 370 (6%) patients, and multivariate analysis revealed that SEMS with high axial force (OR 3.69; $P = .022$) and nonpancreatic cancer (OR 5.52; $P<.001$) were significant risk factors for pancreatitis.[28]

The osmolality of the radiologic contrast material used appears to have no association with the risk of PEP. Studies comparing low-osmolality with high-osmolality contrast media during ERCP show no significant difference in the rate of PEP.[32] Similarly, the benefit of pure cutting current over blended current by reduction of thermal injury during endoscopic sphincterotomy and ampullectomy is controversial.[33–35]

Operator-Related Factors

Operator-related risk factors, such as trainee participation and the case volume and experience of the endoscopist, have been suggested to independently contribute to the risk of PEP, but have been difficult to evaluate. Trainee involvement has been shown to increase the risk of PEP in one study (OR 1.5, 95% CI 1.029–2.057; $P = .03$), which presumably results from traumatic cannulation, prolonging a difficult cannulation, or delivering excess electrosurgical current during sphincterotomy.[14]

Endoscopist case volume is thought to be inversely proportional to the risk of PEP, although most multicenter studies have failed to show this trend. In a prospective multicenter study by Freeman and colleagues,[4] low-volume endoscopists (performing <2 ERCPs per week) had significantly lower success at bile duct cannulation (96.5% vs 91.5%; $P = .0001$), but lower ERCP case volume was not found to be a multivariate risk factor for PEP. Similarly, in a more recent Austrian study, although high case volume (endoscopists performing >50 vs <50 ERCPs per year) was associated with significantly higher success rates (86.9% vs 80.3%; $P<.001$) and lower overall complication rates (10.2% vs 13.6%; $P = .007$), and there was no significant difference in rates of PEP (4.9% vs 5.6%; $P>.05$).[36] This result likely arises because a much higher threshold of case volume is needed to show the impact and the difference in case mix, as low-volume endoscopists tend to perform lower-risk cases.

Although it is difficult to understand the relative contribution and the interactive effect of multiple risk factors, the risk seems to be more than just additive, and a combination of factors can escalate the risk substantially. In one study, the risk of PEP increased from 5% in women with normal serum bilirubin level to 16% with addition of difficult cannulation, with further increase in risk to 42% with addition of suspected SOD as the indication for ERCP.[4] Therefore, careful patient selection, sound endoscopic technique, and tailoring the approach of ERCP to the individual patient are the cornerstones in the prevention of PEP.

METHODS STUDIED TO REDUCE POST–ENDOSCOPIC RETROGRADE CHOLANGIOPANCREATOGRAPHY PANCREATITIS

In addition to avoiding ERCP when the indication is marginal, especially in high-risk patients, several other methods can be used to reduce the risk of PEP. **Box 3**

Box 3
Methods shown to reduce the risk of PEP

- Avoiding unnecessary ERCPs (ie, proper patient selection)
- Guide-wire cannulation technique
- Aggressive hydration
- Early precut (access) sphincterotomy
- Chemoprophylaxis (ie, rectal indomethacin)
- Pancreatic duct stenting, particularly in high-risk cases

---

lists strategies that have been shown to be most effective in reducing PEP. It is important for endoscopists to recognize their limitations, and those less experienced and low-volume providers should consider referring complex cases to high-volume centers. Diagnostic ERCP should be avoided, and alternative imaging techniques such as magnetic resonance cholangiopancreatography (MRCP) and endoscopic ultrasonography (EUS) should be used for excluding obstructive biliary disease.

Guide-Wire Cannulation

Cannulation techniques are recognized to be important in causing PEP. The use of guide-wire–assisted cannulation instead of contrast-guided cannulation to avoid or minimize contrast injection has been shown in some studies to decrease PEP. Contrast-free guide-wire–assisted cannulation is performed either by leading with the guide wire, or inserting the catheter into the papillary orifice and advancing the guide wire without contrast injection. A recent meta-analysis of 12 randomized controlled trials (3450 patients) showed a significant reduction in PEP with a guide-wire–assisted cannulation technique compared with contrast-guided biliary cannulation, with a risk ratio of 0.51 (95% CI 0.32–0.82).[37] In addition, the guide-wire–assisted cannulation technique was associated with greater primary cannulation success (risk ratio 1.07, 95% CI 1.00–1.15), fewer precut sphincterotomies (risk ratio 0.75, 95% CI 0.60–0.95), and no increase in other ERCP-related complications.[37] However, some endoscopists, including the current authors, believe that cannulation without a guide wire is reasonably safe in highly skilled hands and is not associated with increased risks of PEP in comparison with guide-wire cannulation. Many advanced endoscopists use a hybrid of the 2 techniques, using minimal contrast to outline the course of the distal ducts in combination with wire probes, which may avoid dissections or passage of the guide wire outside a side branch of the pancreatic duct.[2] In addition, use of a soft-tipped wire for cannulation may also lower the risk of PEP.

Aggressive Hydration

The use of aggressive periprocedural hydration with lactated Ringer solution also appears to reduce the incidence of PEP. In a recent pilot study of 62 patients, the incidence of PEP was significantly lower (0% vs 17%) in patients randomized to aggressive hydration with lactated Ringer solution (3 mL/kg/h during the procedure, a 20 mL/kg bolus after the procedure, and 3 mL/kg/h for 8 hours after the procedure) compared with patients who received standard hydration with the same solution (1.5 mL/kg/h during and for 8 hours after procedure).[38]

Techniques to Minimize Ampullary Trauma

Efficient and atraumatic technique is central to minimizing the risk of PEP. The risk of PEP can also be reduced by minimizing ampullary trauma by limiting cannulation attempts and using alternative ways of accessing the duct after prolonged cannulation, such as precut or access papillotomy. There has been controversy regarding whether precut techniques increase the risk of PEP, and if the increased risk of PEP is due to the precut papillotomy itself or the prolonged cannulation attempts that often precede its use.[39–43] Comparative studies of precut papillotomy with standard sphincterotomy are difficult to interpret given the difference in indications, settings, experience of the endoscopists, and the frequent combination of precut sphincterotomy with pancreatic stenting.[39–43]

However, there is some evidence to suggest that early precut access, after only 5 to 10 attempts for cannulation, may decrease the risk for PEP compared with persistent attempts at cannulation, which can traumatize the papilla further.[42,44–46] Two previous meta-analyses that included 6 randomized controlled trials comparing early precut papillotomy with persistent attempts at cannulation by a standard approach showed significant reduction in PEP (OR 0.47, 95% CI 0.24–0.91; and rate ratio 0.46, 95% CI 0.23–0.92) when early precut access was obtained.[45,46] A similar trend toward a lower risk of PEP with early use of precut sphincterotomy was also seen in 2 more recent meta-analyses (including 7 randomized controlled trials), although this was not statistically significant (3.9% in the precut sphincterotomy vs 6.1% in the persistent attempts group; OR 0.58, 95% CI 0.32–1.05).[42,47] In addition, early precut strategy was recently shown to substantially reduce the duration of ERCP, which may be clinically beneficial considering the relatively high percentage of elderly and advanced-grade American Society of Anesthesiologists patients.[43]

Chemoprophylaxis

Chemoprophylaxis of PEP has also been suggested and extensively researched in an attempt to prevent or reduce the severity of PEP. Five main targets for chemoprevention include: prevention of intra-acinar trypsinogen activation (protease inhibitors such as gabexate, ulinastatin, nafamostat mesylate)[48]; reduction of pancreatic enzyme secretion (somatostatin and octreotide)[49,50]; relaxation of sphincter of Oddi spasm (nitroglycerin, nifedipine, phosphodiesterase-5 inhibitors)[51–53]; interruption of the inflammatory cascade (nonsteroidal anti-inflammatory drugs [NSAIDs], interleukin-10, corticosteroids, allopurinol, heparin, N-acetylcysteine)[54–60]; and prevention of infection (antibiotics).[61]

However, numerous trials studying a variety of such pharmacologic agents have yielded disappointing or conflicting results; with the important exception of rectal administration of NSAIDs, which have been shown in several randomized controlled trials and meta-analyses to significantly reduce the incidence and severity of PEP.[54–56,62–66] In the largest multicenter, randomized, placebo-controlled, double-blind clinical trial, published in the *New England Journal of Medicine*, 602 patients were randomized to receive a single dose of 100 mg of rectal indomethacin or placebo immediately after ERCP.[55] PEP developed in 9.2% of the indomethacin group and in 16.9% of the placebo group ($P = .005$). Moderate to severe pancreatitis developed in 13 patients (4.4%) in the indomethacin group and in 27 patients (8.8%) in the placebo group ($P = .03$).[55] A recent meta-analysis of 10 randomized controlled trials involving 2269 patients showed that NSAID use decreased the overall incidence of PEP (risk ratio 0.57, 95% CI 0.38–0.86; $P = .007$).[62] Of 10 randomized controlled trials included, indomethacin was administered in 4 studies (rectal route in 3 studies and intraduodenal in 1 study), diclofenac in 5 studies (rectal in 3, oral in 1, and intramuscular in 1), and intravenous valdecoxib was used in 1 study. The pooled number needed to treat was 17. The prophylactic use of NSAIDs was also efficacious in decreasing the incidence of moderate to severe PEP (risk ratio 0.46, 95% CI 0.28–0.75; P = .002). There was no significant difference in the adverse events attributable to NSAIDs.[62]

The mechanism of action of NSAIDs is via potent inhibition of cyclooxygenase, lipoxygenase, and phospholipase-A2 (PLA2) mediated pathways. PLA2 catalyzes the hydrolysis of cell membrane phospholipids, leading to the production of numerous inflammatory mediators such as prostanoids, leukotrienes, kinins, and platelet-activating factor, and is believed to play a critical role in the initial inflammatory cascade in acute pancreatitis.[67–72] Indomethacin and diclofenac are the mostly widely studied and used NSAIDs with similar efficacy in PEP chemoprophylaxis.[73,74] The rectal route in preference to other routes of administration, and administration before (in patients with high preprocedure risk) or immediately after (for patients who move into the high-risk group only during ERCP) the procedure seem to be most effective in preventing PEP.[62,73–75] Based on these data, a good safety profile, and very low cost with one-time dosing, there has been more widespread use of NSAIDs (mainly rectal indomethacin) in patients undergoing ERCP for PEP prevention.

Combination of NSAIDs with other pharmacologic agents or ERCP techniques has also recently been studied in an attempt to achieve higher prophylactic efficacy from synergistic action. A double-blind, placebo-controlled, randomized trial (N = 300) found the combination of rectal indomethacin (100 mg) and sublingual nitrate (5 mg) given before ERCP to be significantly more likely to reduce the incidence of PEP than indomethacin suppository alone (6.7% vs15.3%, respectively; P = .016, risk ratio 0.39, 95% CI 0.18–0.86).[76]

Although mechanistically plausible that stenting and rectal NSAIDs may complement one another by working in completely different ways, a recent network meta-analysis showed that combination of rectal NSAIDs and stents was not superior to either approach alone (NSAIDs plus stents vs NSAIDs alone: OR 1.46, 95% CI 0.79–2.69; NSAIDs plus stents vs stents alone: OR 0.70, 95% CI 0.40–1.20).[77] Post hoc analysis by Elmunzer and colleagues[54] also found rectal indomethacin alone to be more effective for preventing PEP than the combination of indomethacin and pancreatic stents.

Pancreatic Duct Stenting

Pancreatic duct stenting is another intervention that is increasingly used, as it has been shown to reduce the incidence and severity of PEP by mechanically facilitating pancreatic duct drainage by relieving ductal hypertension that develops as a result of transient procedure–induced stenosis of the pancreatic orifice. Several randomized controlled trials and meta-analyses have shown a 60% to 80% reduction in the incidence of pancreatitis with placement of a pancreatic duct stent in high-risk patients.[78–82] A recent meta-analysis, which included 14 randomized controlled trials involving 1541 patients, indeed confirms that placement of prophylactic pancreatic stents is associated with a statistically significant reduction in PEP (RR 0.39, 95% CI 0.29–0.53; P<.001).[83] Subgroup analysis stratified according to the severity of PEP showed that pancreatic stenting was beneficial in patients with mild to moderate PEP (RR 0.45) and in patients with severe PEP (RR 0.26). In addition, subgroup analysis performed according to patient selection demonstrated that stent placement was effective for both high-risk and mixed case groups.[83]

Prophylactic pancreatic stenting is recommended in most patients with difficult cannulation, including double-wire cannulation (whereby a guide wire is left in the pancreatic duct to aid wire cannulation of the common bile duct) and precut sphincterotomy, pancreatic (major or minor) sphincterotomy, pancreatic endotherapy, diagnostic or therapeutic ERCP for suspected or confirmed SOD, history of PEP, balloon dilation of an intact biliary sphincter, and endoscopic ampullectomy.

However, there are a few considerations that the endoscopist must keep in mind when performing pancreatic duct stenting. First, pancreatic duct stenting can be technically challenging and potentially dangerous if attempted but unsuccessful, as it is associated with a high rate of PEP. Attempts at pancreatic duct cannulation may cause increased pancreatic orifice trauma without providing ductal decompression.[56,78,84,85] In addition, pancreatic stents may cause pancreatic ductal or parenchymal injury, with a risk of permanent ductal stenosis and chronic pancreatitis changes over time.[86] Placement of pancreatic stents made of softer materials and the use of smaller-caliber stents (3F or 4F) have been shown to lower the rates of ductal injury in comparison with conventional 5F polyethylene stents; however, 3F pancreatic stents were found to be inferior to the 5F stents for the prevention of PEP in high-risk patients in a recent network meta-analysis.[87]

These prophylactic pancreatic duct stents are not meant to be left in indefinitely, and follow-up abdominal radiography (AXR) must be done to ensure that they have fallen out in a timely fashion (typically within 2–3 weeks). Therefore, when performing pancreatic duct stenting, consideration should also be given to the increased cost and time associated with follow-up AXR to ensure spontaneous passage of the stent, and additional upper endoscopy to remove retained stents in 5% to 10% of patients.[13,88]

Despite these considerations and limited indirect evidence to suggest that NSAIDs are superior to stents for PEP prophylaxis,[54,77] pancreatic stents are routinely placed in all high-risk cases, as prophylactic pancreatic duct stenting has repeatedly been shown to be effective in preventing and reducing the incidence of severe, life-threatening PEP.[83,89,90]

MANAGEMENT OF POST–ENDOSCOPIC RETROGRADE CHOLANGIOPANCREATOGRAPHY PANCREATITIS

Treatment of PEP is similar to that for acute pancreatitis from any other cause: nothing by mouth, aggressive intravenous hydration, adequate pain control, and supportive care, with close monitoring for early recognition of systemic inflammatory response syndrome (SIRS), organ dysfunction, and other complications. As with other causes of acute pancreatitis, lactated Ringer solution is the preferred isotonic crystalloid replacement fluid for aggressive hydration, as it has been shown to decrease SIRS and the severity and complications of pancreatitis in experimental and clinical studies.[91–93] Checking serum amylase or lipase at 4 to 6 hours after the ERCP might predict the development of PEP, and help decide whether the patient would need to be admitted or could be discharged the same day.

SUMMARY

PEP is the most common complication of ERCP; it can be extremely serious and can lead to long-term morbidity and even death. Every effort to minimize this risk should be undertaken. Diagnostic ERCP should be generally avoided, with few exceptions such as when accompanied by sphincter of Oddi manometry. Surrogate imaging with EUS and MRCP is highly accurate, obviating a diagnostic study.

Careful and judicious patient selection is paramount. The endoscopist must exercise meticulous technique, and patients deemed to be at high risk for PEP should receive rectal indomethacin and pancreatic stenting. Aggressive intravenous hydration has also been shown to be beneficial, and the authors administer this routinely. Early recognition of PEP with prompt supportive care and, if appropriate, treatment in the intensive care unit should be provided.

REFERENCES

1. Bakman Y, Freeman ML. Update on biliary and pancreatic sphincterotomy. Curr Opin Gastroenterol 2012;28:420–6.
2. Freeman ML. Complications of endoscopic retrograde cholangiopancreatography: avoidance and management. Gastrointest Endosc Clin N Am 2012;22:567–86.
3. Freeman ML. Adverse outcomes of ERCP. Gastrointest Endosc 2002;56: S273–82.
4. Freeman ML, DiSario JA, Nelson DB, et al. Risk factors for post-ERCP pancreatitis: a prospective, multicenter study. Gastrointest Endosc 2001;54:425–34.
5. Freeman ML, Nelson DB, Sherman S, et al. Complications of endoscopic biliary sphincterotomy. N Engl J Med 1996;335:909–18.
6. Masci E, Toti G, Mariani A, et al. Complications of diagnostic and therapeutic ERCP: a prospective multicenter study. Am J Gastroenterol 2001;96:417–23.
7. Masci E, Mariani A, Curioni S, et al. Risk factors for pancreatitis following endoscopic retrograde cholangiopancreatography: a meta-analysis. Endoscopy 2003;35:830–4.
8. Cotton PB, Lehman G, Vennes J, et al. Endoscopic sphincterotomy complications and their management: an attempt at consensus. Gastrointest Endosc 1991;37: 383–93.
9. Cotton PB, Garrow DA, Gallagher J, et al. Risk factors for complications after ERCP: a multivariate analysis of 11,497 procedures over 12 years. Gastrointest Endosc 2009;70:80–8.
10. Loperfido S, Angelini G, Benedetti G, et al. Major early complications from diagnostic and therapeutic ERCP: a prospective multicenter study. Gastrointest Endosc 1998;48:1–10.
11. Andriulli A, Loperfido S, Napolitano G, et al. Incidence rates of post-ERCP complications: a systematic survey of prospective studies. Am J Gastroenterol 2007; 102:1781–8.
12. Kochar B, Akshintala VS, Afghani E, et al. Incidence, severity, and mortality of post-ERCP pancreatitis: a systematic review by using randomized, controlled trials. Gastrointest Endosc 2014. [Epub ahead of print].
13. Kubiliun NM, Elmunzer BJ. Preventing pancreatitis after endoscopic retrograde cholangiopancreatography. Gastrointest Endosc Clin N Am 2013;23:769–86.
14. Cheng CL, Sherman S, Watkins JL, et al. Risk factors for post-ERCP pancreatitis: a prospective multicenter study. Am J Gastroenterol 2006;101:139–47.
15. Banerjee N, Hilden K, Baron TH, et al. Endoscopic biliary sphincterotomy is not required for transpapillary SEMS placement for biliary obstruction. Dig Dis Sci 2011;56:591–5.
16. Moffatt DC, Cote GA, Avula H, et al. Risk factors for ERCP-related complications in patients with pancreas divisum: a retrospective study. Gastrointest Endosc 2011;73:963–70.
17. Kahaleh M, Freeman M. Prevention and management of post-endoscopic retrograde cholangiopancreatography complications. Clin Endosc 2012;45:305–12.

18. Disario JA, Freeman ML, Bjorkman DJ, et al. Endoscopic balloon dilation compared with sphincterotomy for extraction of bile duct stones. Gastroenterology 2004;127:1291–9.
19. Cheon YK, Cho KB, Watkins JL, et al. Frequency and severity of post-ERCP pancreatitis correlated with extent of pancreatic ductal opacification. Gastrointest Endosc 2007;65:385–93.
20. Watanabe H, Yoneda M, Tominaga K, et al. Comparison between endoscopic papillary balloon dilatation and endoscopic sphincterotomy for the treatment of common bile duct stones. J Gastroenterol 2007;42:56–62.
21. Baron TH, Harewood GC. Endoscopic balloon dilation of the biliary sphincter compared to endoscopic biliary sphincterotomy for removal of common bile duct stones during ERCP: a metaanalysis of randomized, controlled trials. Am J Gastroenterol 2004;99:1455–60.
22. Weinberg BM, Shindy W, Lo S. Endoscopic balloon sphincter dilation (sphincteroplasty) versus sphincterotomy for common bile duct stones. Cochrane Database Syst Rev 2006;(4):CD004890.
23. Heo JH, Kang DH, Jung HJ, et al. Endoscopic sphincterotomy plus large-balloon dilation versus endoscopic sphincterotomy for removal of bile-duct stones. Gastrointest Endosc 2007;66:720–6 [quiz: 768, 771].
24. Misra SP, Dwivedi M. Large-diameter balloon dilation after endoscopic sphincterotomy for removal of difficult bile duct stones. Endoscopy 2008;40:209–13.
25. Feng Y, Zhu H, Chen X, et al. Comparison of endoscopic papillary large balloon dilation and endoscopic sphincterotomy for retrieval of choledocholithiasis: a meta-analysis of randomized controlled trials. J Gastroenterol 2012;47:655–63.
26. Sherman S, Troiano FP, Hawes RH, et al. Sphincter of Oddi manometry: decreased risk of clinical pancreatitis with use of a modified aspirating catheter. Gastrointest Endosc 1990;36:462–6.
27. Cote GA, Kumar N, Ansstas M, et al. Risk of post-ERCP pancreatitis with placement of self-expandable metallic stents. Gastrointest Endosc 2010;72:748–54.
28. Kawakubo K, Isayama H, Nakai Y, et al. Risk factors for pancreatitis following transpapillary self-expandable metal stent placement. Surg Endosc 2012;26:771–6.
29. Kahaleh M, Behm B, Clarke BW, et al. Temporary placement of covered self-expandable metal stents in benign biliary strictures: a new paradigm? (with video). Gastrointest Endosc 2008;67:446–54.
30. Soderlund C, Linder S. Covered metal versus plastic stents for malignant common bile duct stenosis: a prospective, randomized, controlled trial. Gastrointest Endosc 2006;63:986–95.
31. Maranki J, Yeaton P. Prevention of post-ERCP pancreatitis. Curr Gastroenterol Rep 2013;15:352.
32. Mishkin D, Carpenter S, Croffie J, et al. ASGE technology status evaluation report: radiographic contrast media used in ERCP. Gastrointest Endosc 2005;62:480–4.
33. Elta GH, Barnett JL, Wille RT, et al. Pure cut electrocautery current for sphincterotomy causes less post-procedure pancreatitis than blended current. Gastrointest Endosc 1998;47:149–53.
34. Macintosh DG, Love J, Abraham NS. Endoscopic sphincterotomy by using pure-cut electrosurgical current and the risk of post-ERCP pancreatitis: a prospective randomized trial. Gastrointest Endosc 2004;60:551–6.
35. Stefanidis G, Karamanolis G, Viazis N, et al. A comparative study of postendoscopic sphincterotomy complications with various types of electrosurgical current in patients with choledocholithiasis. Gastrointest Endosc 2003;57:192–7.

36. Kapral C, Duller C, Wewalka F, et al. Case volume and outcome of endoscopic retrograde cholangiopancreatography: results of a nationwide Austrian benchmarking project. Endoscopy 2008;40:625–30.

37. Tse F, Yuan Y, Moayyedi P, et al. Guide wire-assisted cannulation for the prevention of post-ERCP pancreatitis: a systematic review and meta-analysis. Endoscopy 2013;45:605–18.

38. Buxbaum J, Yan A, Yeh K, et al. Aggressive hydration with lactated Ringer's solution reduces pancreatitis after endoscopic retrograde cholangiopancreatography. Clin Gastroenterol Hepatol 2014;12:303–7.e1.

39. Misra SP. Pre-cut sphincterotomy: does the timing matter? Gastrointest Endosc 2009;69:480–3.

40. Tham TC, Vandervoort J. Needle-knife sphincterotomy and post-ERCP pancreatitis: time to lower the threshold for the needle? Gastrointest Endosc 2010;71:272–4.

41. Cotton PB. It's not the precut; it's the why done and who by. Gastrointest Endosc 2010;72:1114 [author reply:1114].

42. Choudhary A, Winn J, Siddique S, et al. Effect of precut sphincterotomy on post-endoscopic retrograde cholangiopancreatography pancreatitis: a systematic review and meta-analysis. World J Gastroenterol 2014;20:4093–101.

43. Lopes L, Dinis-Ribeiro M, Rolanda C. Early precut fistulotomy for biliary access: time to change the paradigm of "the later, the better?". Gastrointest Endosc 2014; 80(4):634–41.

44. Zhu JH, Liu Q, Zhang DQ, et al. Evaluation of early precut with needle-knife in difficult biliary cannulation during ERCP. Dig Dis Sci 2013;58:3606–10.

45. Cennamo V, Fuccio L, Zagari RM, et al. Can early precut implementation reduce endoscopic retrograde cholangiopancreatography-related complication risk? Meta-analysis of randomized controlled trials. Endoscopy 2010;42:381–8.

46. Gong B, Hao L, Bie L, et al. Does precut technique improve selective bile duct cannulation or increase post-ERCP pancreatitis rate? A meta-analysis of randomized controlled trials. Surg Endosc 2010;24:2670–80.

47. Navaneethan U, Konjeti R, Venkatesh PG, et al. Early precut sphincterotomy and the risk of endoscopic retrograde cholangiopancreatography related complications: an updated meta-analysis. World J Gastrointest Endosc 2014;6:200–8.

48. Yuhara H, Ogawa M, Kawaguchi Y, et al. Pharmacologic prophylaxis of post-endoscopic retrograde cholangiopancreatography pancreatitis: protease inhibitors and NSAIDs in a meta-analysis. J Gastroenterol 2014;49:388–99.

49. Omata F, Deshpande G, Tokuda Y, et al. Meta-analysis: somatostatin or its long-acting analogue, octreotide, for prophylaxis against post-ERCP pancreatitis. J Gastroenterol 2010;45:885–95.

50. Zhao LN, Yu T, Li CQ, et al. Somatostatin administration prior to ERCP is effective in reducing the risk of post-ERCP pancreatitis in high-risk patients. Exp Ther Med 2014;8:509–14.

51. Prat F, Amaris J, Ducot B, et al. Nifedipine for prevention of post-ERCP pancreatitis: a prospective, double-blind randomized study. Gastrointest Endosc 2002; 56:202–8.

52. Oh HC, Cheon YK, Cho YD, et al. Use of udenafil is not associated with a reduction in post-ERCP pancreatitis: results of a randomized, placebo-controlled, multicenter trial. Gastrointest Endosc 2011;74:556–62.

53. Nojgaard C, Hornum M, Elkjaer M, et al. Does glyceryl nitrate prevent post-ERCP pancreatitis? A prospective, randomized, double-blind, placebo-controlled multicenter trial. Gastrointest Endosc 2009;69:e31–7.

54. Elmunzer BJ, Higgins PD, Saini SD, et al. Does rectal indomethacin eliminate the need for prophylactic pancreatic stent placement in patients undergoing high-risk ERCP? Post hoc efficacy and cost-benefit analyses using prospective clinical trial data. Am J Gastroenterol 2013;108:410–5.

55. Elmunzer BJ, Scheiman JM, Lehman GA, et al. A randomized trial of rectal indomethacin to prevent post-ERCP pancreatitis. N Engl J Med 2012;366: 1414–22.

56. Elmunzer BJ, Waljee AK. Can rectal NSAIDs replace prophylactic pancreatic stent placement for the prevention of post-ERCP pancreatitis? Gastroenterology 2014;146:313–5 [discussion: 315].

57. Bai Y, Gao J, Shi X, et al. Prophylactic corticosteroids do not prevent post-ERCP pancreatitis: a meta-analysis of randomized controlled trials. Pancreatology 2008;8:504–9.

58. Zheng M, Chen Y, Bai J, et al. Meta-analysis of prophylactic allopurinol use in post-endoscopic retrograde cholangiopancreatography pancreatitis. Pancreas 2008;37:247–53.

59. Li S, Cao G, Chen X, et al. Low-dose heparin in the prevention of post endoscopic retrograde cholangiopancreatography pancreatitis: a systematic review and meta-analysis. Eur J Gastroenterol Hepatol 2012;24:477–81.

60. Katsinelos P, Kountouras J, Paroutoglou G, et al. Intravenous N-acetylcysteine does not prevent post-ERCP pancreatitis. Gastrointest Endosc 2005;62:105–11.

61. Raty S, Sand J, Pulkkinen M, et al. Post-ERCP pancreatitis: reduction by routine antibiotics. J Gastrointest Surg 2001;5:339–45 [discussion: 345].

62. Ding X, Chen M, Huang S, et al. Nonsteroidal anti-inflammatory drugs for prevention of post-ERCP pancreatitis: a meta-analysis. Gastrointest Endosc 2012;76: 1152–9.

63. Sotoudehmanesh R, Khatibian M, Kolahdoozan S, et al. Indomethacin may reduce the incidence and severity of acute pancreatitis after ERCP. Am J Gastroenterol 2007;102:978–83.

64. Cheon YK, Cho KB, Watkins JL, et al. Efficacy of diclofenac in the prevention of post-ERCP pancreatitis in predominantly high-risk patients: a randomized double-blind prospective trial. Gastrointest Endosc 2007;66:1126–32.

65. Senol A, Saritas U, Demirkan H. Efficacy of intramuscular diclofenac and fluid replacement in prevention of post-ERCP pancreatitis. World J Gastroenterol 2009;15:3999–4004.

66. Otsuka T, Kawazoe S, Nakashita S, et al. Low-dose rectal diclofenac for prevention of post-endoscopic retrograde cholangiopancreatography pancreatitis: a randomized controlled trial. J Gastroenterol 2012;47:912–7.

67. Folch E, Closa D, Prats N, et al. Leukotriene generation and neutrophil infiltration after experimental acute pancreatitis. Inflammation 1998;22:83–93.

68. Vollmar B, Waldner H, Schmand J, et al. Release of arachidonic acid metabolites during acute pancreatitis in pigs. Scand J Gastroenterol 1989;24: 1253–64.

69. Sherman S, Alazmi WM, Lehman GA, et al. Evaluation of recombinant platelet-activating factor acetylhydrolase for reducing the incidence and severity of post-ERCP acute pancreatitis. Gastrointest Endosc 2009;69:462–72.

70. Yamamoto K, Shinomura Y, Tojo H, et al. Serum pancreatic phospholipase A2 and prophospholipase A2 in acute pancreatitis and after endoscopic retrograde pancreatography. Gastroenterol Jpn 1993;28:679–86.

71. Zhang KJ, Zhang DL, Jiao XL, et al. Effect of phospholipase A2 silencing on acute experimental pancreatitis. Eur Rev Med Pharmacol Sci 2013;17:3279–84.

72. Kahl S, Mayer J, Schuette K, et al. Effect of procainhydrochloride on phospholipase A2 catalytic activity in sodium taurocholate-induced acute experimental pancreatitis in rats. Dig Dis 2010;28:373–8.
73. Puig I, Calvet X, Baylina M, et al. How and when should NSAIDs be used for preventing post-ERCP pancreatitis? A systematic review and meta-analysis. PLoS One 2014;9:e92922.
74. Sethi S, Sethi N, Wadhwa V, et al. A meta-analysis on the role of rectal diclofenac and indomethacin in the prevention of post-endoscopic retrograde cholangiopancreatography pancreatitis. Pancreas 2014;43:190–7.
75. Ahmad D, Lopez KT, Esmadi MA, et al. The effect of indomethacin in the prevention of post-endoscopic retrograde cholangiopancreatography pancreatitis: a meta-analysis. Pancreas 2014;43:338–42.
76. Sotoudehmanesh R, Eloubeidi MA, Asgari AA, et al. A randomized trial of rectal indomethacin and sublingual nitrates to prevent post-ERCP pancreatitis. Am J Gastroenterol 2014;109:903–9.
77. Akbar A, Abu Dayyeh BK, Baron TH, et al. Rectal nonsteroidal anti-inflammatory drugs are superior to pancreatic duct stents in preventing pancreatitis after endoscopic retrograde cholangiopancreatography: a network meta-analysis. Clin Gastroenterol Hepatol 2013;11:778–83.
78. Bhatia V, Ahuja V, Acharya SK, et al. A randomized controlled trial of valdecoxib and glyceryl trinitrate for the prevention of post-ERCP pancreatitis. J Clin Gastroenterol 2011;45:170–6.
79. Fazel A, Quadri A, Catalano MF, et al. Does a pancreatic duct stent prevent post-ERCP pancreatitis? A prospective randomized study. Gastrointest Endosc 2003;57:291–4.
80. Singh P, Das A, Isenberg G, et al. Does prophylactic pancreatic stent placement reduce the risk of post-ERCP acute pancreatitis? A meta-analysis of controlled trials. Gastrointest Endosc 2004;60:544–50.
81. Tarnasky PR. Mechanical prevention of post-ERCP pancreatitis by pancreatic stents: results, techniques, and indications. JOP 2003;4:58–67.
82. Choudhary A, Bechtold ML, Arif M, et al. Pancreatic stents for prophylaxis against post-ERCP pancreatitis: a meta-analysis and systematic review. Gastrointest Endosc 2011;73:275–82.
83. Mazaki T, Mado K, Masuda H, et al. Prophylactic pancreatic stent placement and post-ERCP pancreatitis: an updated meta-analysis. J Gastroenterol 2014;49:343–55.
84. Freeman ML. Prevention of post-ERCP pancreatitis: pharmacologic solution or patient selection and pancreatic stents? Gastroenterology 2003;124:1977–80.
85. Freeman ML, Overby C, Qi D. Pancreatic stent insertion: consequences of failure and results of a modified technique to maximize success. Gastrointest Endosc 2004;59:8–14.
86. Kozarek RA. Pancreatic stents can induce ductal changes consistent with chronic pancreatitis. Gastrointest Endosc 1990;36:93–5.
87. Afghani E, Akshintala VS, Khashab MA, et al. 5-Fr vs. 3-Fr pancreatic stents for the prevention of post-ERCP pancreatitis in high-risk patients: a systematic review and network meta-analysis. Endoscopy 2014;46:573–80.
88. Chahal P, Tarnasky PR, Petersen BT, et al. Short 5Fr vs long 3Fr pancreatic stents in patients at risk for post-endoscopic retrograde cholangiopancreatography pancreatitis. Clin Gastroenterol Hepatol 2009;7:834–9.
89. Arain MA, Freeman ML. Pharmacologic prophylaxis alone is not adequate to prevent post-ERCP pancreatitis. Am J Gastroenterol 2014;109:910–2.

90. Freeman ML. Pancreatic stents for prevention of post-ERCP pancreatitis: the evidence is irrefutable. J Gastroenterol 2014;49:369–70.
91. Tenner S, Baillie J, DeWitt J, et al. American College of Gastroenterology guideline: management of acute pancreatitis. Am J Gastroenterol 2013;108:1400–15, 16.
92. Hoque R, Farooq A, Ghani A, et al. Lactate reduces liver and pancreatic injury in Toll-like receptor- and inflammasome-mediated inflammation via GPR81-mediated suppression of innate immunity. Gastroenterology 2014;146:1763–74.
93. Wu BU, Hwang JQ, Gardner TH, et al. Lactated Ringer's solution reduces systemic inflammation compared with saline in patients with acute pancreatitis. Clin Gastroenterol Hepatol 2011;9:710–7.e1.

Achieving Hemostasis and the Risks Associated with Therapy

Nayantara Coelho Prabhu, MBBS, Louis M. Wong Kee Song, MD*

KEYWORDS

- Clips • Endoscopic band ligation • Gastrointestinal bleeding • Hemostatic spray
- Hemostasis • Peptic ulcer bleeding • Perforation • Thermal coagulation

KEY POINTS

- The major adverse events attributed to endoscopic hemostasis include precipitation of uncontrollable bleeding and perforation.
- The effective and safe application of endoscopic hemostasis necessitates a working knowledge of the various hemostatic tools available and recognition of pitfalls of endotherapy based on the location and characteristics of the targeted lesion.

Videos demonstrating endoscopic hemostasis accompany this article at
http://www.giendo.theclinics.com/

INTRODUCTION

Despite the declining trend in admission for acute gastrointestinal (GI) bleeding,[1] the condition still remains a common cause for hospitalization and a source of significant morbidity and mortality.[2] Endoscopic diagnosis and therapy are an integral part of the management algorithm for acute GI bleeding. A variety of hemostatic tools are at the disposal of the endoscopist, and a working knowledge of these devices is essential for their safe and effective use. Herein, the authors highlight the applications and caveats of endoscopic hemostasis from a device perspective.

PITFALLS OF ENDOSCOPIC HEMOSTASIS

Determinants for a successful outcome include the availability and appropriate selection of particular devices for hemostasis, the experience and skill of the operator, and the suitability of the targeted lesion for endoscopic therapy. It is imperative to recognize potential pitfalls of endotherapy based on the location and features of the

Division of Gastroenterology and Hepatology, Mayo Clinic, 200 1st Street Southwest, Rochester, MN 55905, USA
* Corresponding author.
E-mail address: wong.louis@mayo.edu

Gastrointest Endoscopy Clin N Am 25 (2015) 123–145
http://dx.doi.org/10.1016/j.giec.2014.09.012
1052-5157/15/$ – see front matter © 2015 Elsevier Inc. All rights reserved.

bleeding lesion. Failure to recognize potentially problematic lesions can result in serious adverse events, such as precipitation of uncontrollable bleeding and perforation, during attempted endoscopic hemostasis.

Lesion Location

Endoscopic therapy for lesions in the territories of the left gastric artery (LGA) and gastroduodenal artery (GDA) needs careful consideration because these lesions are usually fed by large-caliber vessels. The problem is further compounded by the endoscopic difficulty in accessing these lesions. A salvage plan consisting of angiographic and/or surgical intervention needs to be established before attempted endotherapy in the event of iatrogenic uncontrollable bleeding. The LGA and its tributaries course along the proximal lesser curvature of the stomach. This area is also a technically difficult area to access with the endoscope in both direct and retroflexed positions. Inconspicuous lesions, such as a small Dieulafoy lesion, can hide behind the shaft of the retroflexed endoscope. Deeply penetrating ulcers with high-risk stigmata (HRS) of recent hemorrhage (eg, dense adherent clot) and large Dieulafoy lesions (>2 mm) arising from the main LGA are prone to brisk bleeding and are not usually amenable to standard endoscopic therapy, such as coaptive coagulation. Prophylactic radiologic embolization may be appropriate for these lesions because of the high incidence of potentially life-threatening rebleeding. Placement of through-the-scope (TTS) clips adjacent to the bleeding site can serve as fluoroscopic markers to facilitate subsequent supraselective angiographic embolization.

The GDA usually arises from the common hepatic artery, supplies the proximal duodenum, and can be a source of significant bleeding in the setting of peptic ulcer disease (PUD). Access to ulcers on the posteroinferior duodenal wall and treatment of underlying bleeding stigmata can be challenging because of restricted visualization at the duodenal angle and an unstable endoscope position, especially if the bulb is short and edematous. Cap-assisted hemostasis can potentially remedy this situation (see later discussion). In addition, culprit vessels arising from the GDA can be large and difficult to treat adequately with conventional TTS clips and contact thermal probes. If therapy is entertained, a duodenal ulcer with a dense adherent clot should undergo large-volume epinephrine injection before clot removal by cold snare guillotine, followed by definitive therapy for the underlying bleeding stigmata, as appropriate (Video 1). In general, readily accessible visible vessels (VV) 2 mm or less in size are amenable to contact coagulation (10F thermal probe) or TTS clip placement (**Fig. 1**). Newer devices, such as the over-the-scope clip (OTSC), may be effective at managing lesions with bleeding vessels greater than 2 mm in size, although OTSC data for this indication are scant (**Fig. 2**). For lesions in which conventional endoscopic hemostasis is thought to be too risky (eg, VV >2 mm) and the risk of rebleeding without endotherapy is high, prophylactic angiographic embolization is an option. As previously mentioned, placement of TTS clips close to the bleeding point can assist as fluoroscopic markers for supraselective coil embolization (**Fig. 3**).

Other locations where careful endotherapy is warranted include the thin-walled colon (in particular, cecum and diverticular dome) and the small bowel, especially when contact thermal probes are used. Distention of these segments should be curtailed to avoid thinning the wall even further before application of thermal therapy in order to minimize the risk of perforation.

Lesion Features

For shallow bleeding peptic ulcers with HRS, endoscopic management consisting of thermal or mechanical (clip) therapy, with or without epinephrine injection, is typically

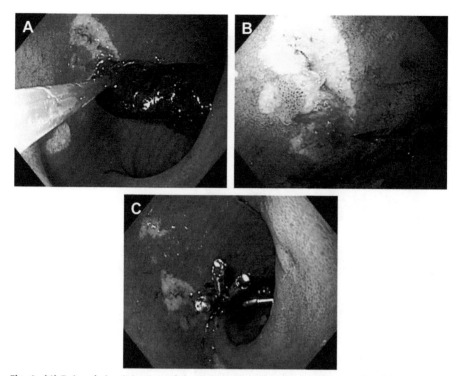

Fig. 1. (*A*) Epinephrine injection of duodenal ulcer with dense adherent clot. (*B*) VV (*arrow*) visualized following clot removal. (*C*) Definitive hemostasis with clip placement.

effective.[3] Deeply penetrating ulcers, however, represent a therapeutic challenge. It is important to carefully assess the surrounding of a deceptively small, pigmented protuberance or VV in the base of a penetrating ulcer, as this may represent only the tip of the iceberg. The presence of transmitted pulsations at the base of the protuberance suggests a much larger feeding vessel (Video 2) or even a pseudoaneurysm. These lesions are not suitable for endoscopic therapy.

The use of TTS clips to target a nonbleeding VV in a large fibrotic ulcer base is often ineffective and can result in torrential bleeding caused by avulsion of the vessel during attempted clip placement. Moreover, clip closure of the entire ulcerated defect is

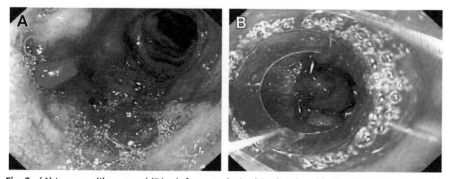

Fig. 2. (*A*) Large-caliber vessel (Dieulafoy-type lesion) in duodenal bulb. (*B*) OTSC placement.

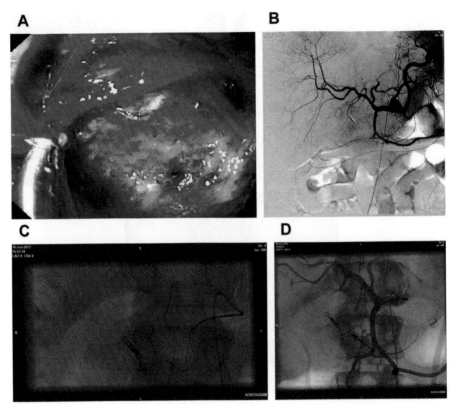

Fig. 3. (*A*) Deeply penetrating duodenal ulcer with placement of clip adjacent large VV. (*B*) Mesenteric angiogram after clip placement. (*C*) Supraselective catheterization of bleeding vessel aided by visualization of endoscopically placed clip. (*D*) Supraselective coil embolization of feeding vessel (*arrow*).

unlikely to be successful because the clips may not have sufficient compression force to collapse the indurated base. In this setting, a contact thermal probe may be more appropriate for a vessel less than 2 mm in size, although the penetrating nature of the ulcer increases the risk of perforation during coaptive coagulation.

Endoscopic suturing may be able to oversew these lesions, but experience with this approach is limited.

PRACTICAL POINTERS FOR ENDOSCOPIC HEMOSTASIS
Water Irrigation and Immersion

During endoscopy, areas accumulating fresh blood and clots should be washed vigorously, as they herald a potential underlying or adjacent bleeding site. A pedal-activated water jet irrigation device coupled to the endoscope is especially useful for removing adherent material from the mucosa and to precisely pinpoint the bleeding site for targeted therapy. Examination under water immersion can also be helpful in identifying the nature and location of the bleeding lesion that is otherwise difficult to visualize (Video 3).

Cap-Assisted Hemostasis

Placement of a transparent hard cap (similar to a band ligation cap) at the tip of the endoscope can assist in delivering hemostasis to segments of the gut that are otherwise difficult to access. These areas include the distal tangential aspect of the cardia, the duodenal angle, a narrowed and angulated sigmoid colon, the distal rectum, and behind folds (Video 4), among others. The cap provides a working window for optimal visualization of the lesion and passage of accessories, aids in securing a stable endoscope position, and can tamponade the bleeding point while hemostatic devices are being readied (Video 5).

String-Assisted Retroflexion

A lesion situated high in the fundus may be difficult to access despite maximal retroflexion of the endoscope. The technique of string-assisted retroflexion involves tying a sufficiently long and strong suture with its knot at the distal tip and on the inner bent portion of the retroflexed endoscope (**Fig. 4**). With the endoscope retroflexed in the stomach, countertraction applied to the string at the mouth will accentuate the bending angle of the endoscope and enable potential therapy for these difficult-to-access fundal lesions (Video 6). The hemostatic accessory should exit the working channel of the endoscope before retroflexion because passage of the device is hindered by the tightly retroflexed configuration of the endoscope.

HEMOSTATIC TECHNIQUES
Injection Therapies

Epinephrine
Epinephrine is commonly injected in a 1:10,000 dilution for hemostasis of nonvariceal bleeding lesions. Its mechanisms of action consist of local vasoconstriction and volume tamponade of the vessel. Because its effects are transient, epinephrine should be combined with a more definitive therapy for hemostasis, such as coaptive coagulation or clip placement.[4]

In the setting of bleeding peptic ulcers, epinephrine should be injected before removal of an adherent clot or when active bleeding is present. Epinephrine may stop or slow active arterial bleeding (spurting) sufficiently to improve visibility and enable precise targeting of the bleeding point. For a nonbleeding VV, injections 1 to 3 mm away from (not directly into) the vessel should be performed. Although a 4-quadrant injection around the bleeding point is desirable, it is important to avoid injection in areas whereby creation of a submucosal bleb lifts the target site away from view and compromises access to further therapy. Conversely, injection can be performed in a manner that improves lesion access for definitive therapy (Video 7). For peptic ulcers,

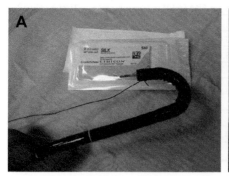
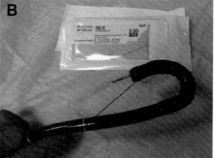

Fig. 4. (*A*) String-assisted retroflexion. (*B*) Countertraction on the string accentuates the bending angle of the endoscope for accessing high fundal lesions.

large-volume (>10 mL) is better than small-volume (≤10 mL) epinephrine injection in reducing the rate of recurrent bleeding[5]; it may also decrease the risk of brisk bleeding during clot removal.

Epinephrine injection can cause clinically significant tachyarrhythmias and hypertension, especially when injected into segments of the gut where first-pass metabolism is bypassed (eg, esophagus). In those areas, injection of a more dilute epinephrine solution (eg, 1:100,000) should be considered. Epinephrine injection should be avoided in the presence of active ischemic cardiomyopathy, and an equally effective tamponade effect can be achieved with the injection of normal saline in this setting.

The vasospasm induced by epinephrine injection can be quite pronounced and sometimes interferes with localization of the culprit vessel during a salvage angiographic procedure. In cases when control of bleeding is not achieved during endoscopy, a hemostatic clip should be placed as close as possible to the bleeding site to guide the interventional angiography instead of repeated overinjections of epinephrine.

Sclerosants

Sclerosing agents induce vascular thrombosis leading to obliteration. They have been used primarily for the treatment of variceal hemorrhage, including esophageal and gastric and ectopic varices.[6,7] Sclerotherapy is generally used as second-line therapy when endoscopic band ligation (EBL) is not feasible or fails in the setting of active esophageal variceal hemorrhage. Several sclerosants are available for use and are of comparable efficacy. However, the maximum volume injected per site and per session varies among the sclerosants because of the differences in potency and the degree of tissue injury (**Table 1**).[6] The selection of a particular sclerosing agent is largely based on personal preference and availability.

A 23-gauge injection needle is typically used, and injections can be directed into the varix (intravariceal) or adjacent to the varix (paravariceal). Intravariceal injections may be associated with fewer adverse events than the paravariceal approach, although the intended injection technique may not be straightforward, particularly in the setting of a bloody field of view.[8] Sclerosants are rarely used for nonvariceal lesions because of the unpredictable depth of injury and availability of equally effective and safer alternatives.

A host of local and systemic adverse events have been described in as many as 25% of patients who undergo variceal sclerotherapy. These events include chest

| Table 1 | | | |
| **Sclerosing agents** | | | |
Agents	Volume per Injection Site (mL)*	Volume per Session (mL)^	Relative Tissue Injury$
Fatty acid derivatives			
Ethanolamine oleate (5%)	1.5–5.0	20	+++
Sodium morrhuate (5%)	0.5–5.0	15	+++
Synthetic agents			
Sodium tetradecyl sulfate (1% & 3%)	1–2	10	++
Polidocanol (0.5%–3%)	1–2	20	+
Alcohols			
Ethanol (99.5%)	0.3–0.5	4–5	++++
Phenol (3%)	3–5	30	+

* Recommended dose per injection site.
^ Maximum volume recommended per session.
$ Least (+) to most (++++) potency for tissue injury.

pain, fever, pleural effusions, sclerotherapy-induced ulcer bleeding, symptomatic strictures, mediastinitis, fistulas (**Fig. 5**), perforations, mesenteric or portal vein thrombosis, spontaneous bacterial peritonitis, and sepsis, among others.[9] Bacteremia occurs in up to 50% of patients undergoing sclerotherapy, and prophylactic antibiotics should be administered in cirrhotic patients presenting with GI bleeding, regardless of sclerotherapy.

Tissue adhesives

Cyanoacrylates are a class of synthetic glues that polymerize rapidly on contact with blood and are used primarily for the treatment of gastric variceal hemorrhage.[10,11] Two commonly used agents in endoscopy include n-butyl-2 cyanoacrylate (BCA) (Indermil, Covidien, Mansfield, MA) and 2-octyl cyanoacrylate (OCA) (Dermabond, Ethicon, Somerville, NJ). Both agents are used off label in the United States for the purpose of gastric variceal obliteration. A standardized institutional protocol for intravariceal cyanoacrylate injection may enhance the efficacy and safety of the procedure,[12] although variations in technique exist based on the type of cyanoacrylate used and local expertise (**Table 2**). BCA is generally mixed with an oily contrast agent (Lipiodol, Guerbet LLC, Bloomington, IN) in a 1:1 ratio to prevent premature solidification of the glue in the injection catheter and needle impaction in the varix. In contrast, OCA must be injected undiluted to minimize the risk of glue embolization caused by its longer ester chain linked to the main compound, which delays its polymerization. Relative to BCA, a larger injection volume of OCA is needed to achieve similar vascular occlusion.[13] A 21-gauge injection catheter with an 8-mm-long needle is recommended to ensure intravariceal puncture. The tip and working channel of the endoscope should be lubricated with Lipiodol or silicone oil to prevent glue adhesion and potential irreparable damage to the endoscope. Suction should also be avoided during the injection procedure. Patients and staff should wear protective eyewear during the procedure.

Following priming of the injection catheter with Lipiodol, 1 to 2 mL of the BCA-Lipiodol mixture is injected into the gastric varix per puncture site followed immediately by an injection of approximately 1 mL of sterile water, equivalent to the catheter's dead space. For OCA, the injection catheter is primed with normal saline instead of Lipiodol. OCA can be injected slowly in 1-mL aliquots[14] or continuously at a rate of 1 mL over 15 to 20 seconds until resistance is met during the syringe push; this typically occurs after 2 to 3 mL of OCA has been injected into the varix.[15] Saline solution

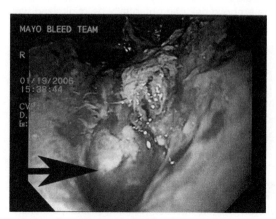

Fig. 5. Sclerotherapy-induced esophago-pleural fistula (*arrow*).

Table 2
BCA versus OCA injection for gastric variceal hemorrhage

	BCA	OCA
Mixed with Lipiodol	Yes>no	No
Glue-Lipiodol ratio	~1:1	Not applicable
Injection volume per puncture site (mL)	1–2	2–4
Maximum volume injected per session (mL)	≤5	≤10

(~1 mL) is then used to flush the injection catheter while it is being retracted from the punctured site. Several sites can be injected per treatment session, aiming for complete variceal obturation at the initial session. To avoid instrument damage, the injection catheter should not be withdrawn through the working channel of the endoscope. Instead, the catheter tip is left trailing the tip of the endoscope by several centimeters. On endoscope withdrawal, the catheter is sectioned at the entrance port of the working channel and pulled from the tip of the endoscope (Video 8).

Cyanoacrylate is more effective than sclerotherapy and EBL and as effective as transjugular intrahepatic portosystemic shunt (TIPS) in controlling and preventing gastric variceal hemorrhage.[16–18] Transient low-grade fever may occur as a result of a foreign-body response to cyanoacrylate, and prophylactic antibiotics should be administered before glue injection. Serious adverse events (eg, pulmonary embolism and stroke) from glue embolization (**Fig. 6**) are of major concern, although the incidence for clinically significant embolic events was low (0.7%) in a large retrospective study encompassing 753 patients.[19] In another study whereby chest computed tomography (CT) was performed in all patients who underwent variceal cyanoacrylate injection, a high incidence of pulmonary glue embolism (47%) was found, albeit subclinical in all patients. This finding is noteworthy, especially given that such a small volume of glue (1 mL) was injected per session.[20] Additional adverse events related to cyanoacrylate injection include sepsis, fistulas, ulcer bleeding at the puncture site, and needle entrapment in the varix.[12]

Before consideration of glue injection for gastric varices, a dynamic CT scan is recommended to determine the presence of spontaneous large splenorenal or gastrorenal shunts (GRS). These shunts are major routes through which glue embolization occurs. The presence of intracardiac or intrapulmonary shunts, as assessed by contrast echocardiogram, also heightens the risk for systemic glue embolization.[21] Although the embolic risk can potentially be minimized with the introduction

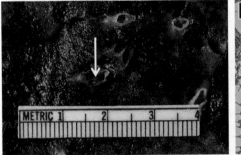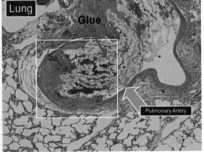

Fig. 6. Intravariceal cyanoacrylate injection resulting in fatal pulmonary glue embolization (*white arrow*) Embolic glue material in vessel. H and E stain, magnification 40×.

of novel techniques, such as endoscopic ultrasound–guided coil/glue injection and the combined approach of endoscopic cyanoacrylate injection with angiographic balloon occlusion of the GRS (**Fig. 7**), further assessment of these modalities is warranted.[22–24]

The experience regarding injection of thrombin or fibrin sealants for gastric variceal hemorrhage is limited.[25] Embolic adverse events have not been described, but leakage of thrombin into the systemic circulation via a GRS could potentially induce disseminated intravascular coagulation or pulmonary embolism.

Thermal Modalities

Bipolar and heater probes

Contact thermal modalities, such as bipolar and heater probes, enable coaptive coagulation and sealing of blood vessels. The probes are available in sizes of 7F and 10F to fit diagnostic and therapeutic working channels, respectively. In the setting of acute bleeding, therapeutic endoscopes should be used, when feasible, for better suction capability and to accommodate the larger thermal probes. Lesions with bleeding vessels up to 2 mm in size can be treated effectively with the 10F probes, including peptic ulcers, Dieulafoy lesions, Mallory-Weiss tears, diverticular bleeding, postpolypectomy bleeding, and vascular ectasias.

In general, bleeding peptic ulcers and Dieulafoy lesions require higher power settings, firmer probe-tissue contact pressure, and longer duration of application, whereas lesions in the small bowel and colon, such as angioectasias, necessitate lower power settings, lighter probe-tissue contact pressure, and shorter pulse duration to minimize the risk of perforation (**Table 3**).[26] The built-in water jet irrigation is a useful feature to identify the bleeding point in the setting of active bleeding and to lessen probe-tissue stickiness and ease separation of the probe from the coagulated lesion. A shallow depression with coagulum formation is the desired end result (**Fig. 8**).

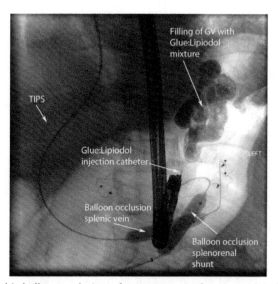

Fig. 7. Angiographic balloon occlusion of portosystemic shunts to minimize systemic glue embolization during endoscopic cyanoacrylate injection of bleeding gastric varices following failed TIPS.

Table 3
Suggested settings for thermal therapies of selected nonvariceal bleeding lesions

Thermal Modalities	Upper GI Lesions				Lower GI Lesions				
	PUD	Dieulafoy	MWT	GAVE	Diverticular Bleeding	Postpolypectomy Bleeding	Angioectasia§	Focal Ulcer	Cancer
Bipolar									
Probe size* (large 10F or small 7F)	Large	Large	Large or small	Large	Large>small	Large>small	Large>small	Large>small	Large>small
Power (W)	15–20	15–20	12–15	15	12–15	12–15	12–15	12–15	12–15
Application duration (s)**	7–10	7–10	3–5	3–5	2–4	2–4	2–4	2–4	2–4
No. of applications (on average)	Variable (1–5)	Variable (1–5)	Variable (1–5)	Multiple	Variable (1–5)	Variable (1–5)	Variable (1–5)	Variable (1–5)	Variable (1–5)
Tamponade/probe-tissue pressure	Firm	Firm	Moderate	Moderate	Light-moderate	Light-moderate	Light-moderate	Moderate	Moderate
End point	Bleed stops; white coagulum; cavitation	Bleed stops; white coagulum; cavitation	Bleed stops; white coagulum	Bleed stops; white coagulum	Bleed stops; white coagulum	Bleed stops	Bleed stops; white coagulum	Bleed stops	Bleed stops
Heater Probe									
Probe size* (large 10F or small 7F)	Large	Large	Large or small	Large	Large>small	Large>small	Large>small	Large>small	Large>small

Power (J)	30	30	15	15	15	15	15	15	15
Application duration (s)	Preset	Preset	Preset	Preset	Preset	Preset	Preset	Preset	Preset
No. of applications	Variable (1–5)	Variable (1–5)	Variable (1–5)	Multiple	Variable (1–5)	Variable (1–5)	Variable (1–5)	Variable (1–5)	Variable (1–5)
Tamponade/probe-tissue pressure	Firm	Firm	Moderate	Moderate	Light-moderate	Light-moderate	Light-moderate	Moderate	Moderate
End point	Bleed stops; white coagulum; cavitation	Bleed stops; white coagulum; cavitation	Bleed stops; white coagulum	Bleed stops; white coagulum	Bleed stops; white coagulum	Bleed stops	Bleed stops; white coagulum	Bleed stops	Bleed stops
APC &									
Power (W)	N/A	N/A	30–45	35–60	30–45	30–45	30–45	30–45	30–45
Argon gas flow rate (L/min)	—	—	1	1	1	1	1	1	1
Probe-to-tissue distance (mm)	1–2	1–2	1–2	1–2	1–2	1–2	1–2	1–2	1–2
End point	—	—	Bleed stops; coagulum	White coagulum	Bleed stops; white coagulum	Bleed stops	Bleed stops; white coagulum	Bleed stops	Bleed stops

Abbreviations: APC, argon plasma coagulation; GAVE, gastric antral vascular ectasia; MWT, mallory weiss tear; NA, not applicable; PUD, peptic ulcer disease.
* Large probe preferred if therapeutic channel endoscope utilized.
** Duration of application before removing the probe.
$ Initiate coagulation at periphery of the lesion, then toward its center.
& Coaptive (contact) coagulation preferred over APC for bleeding PUD and Dieulafoy lesion.

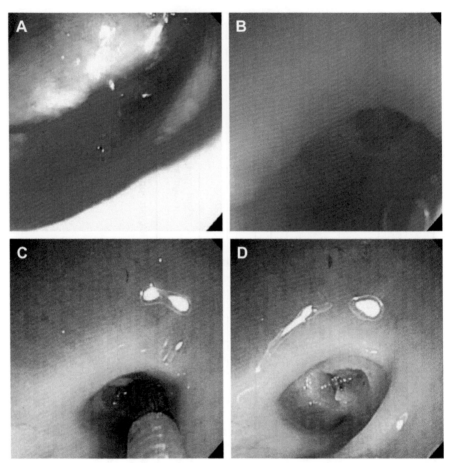

Fig. 8. (*A*) Active arterial bleeding during mucosal resection. (*B*) VV identified under water immersion. (*C*) Heater probe coagulation of VV. (*D*) Appearance after therapy.

Precipitation or inability to control active bleeding occurs when targeting a vessel larger than the probe itself or due to technical deficiencies (eg, insufficient tamponade pressure). Perforations can occur from excessive force application, particularly in thin-walled segments of the gut, and during coaptive coagulation of a deeply penetrating ulcer. If recognized immediately, these small iatrogenic perforations may be amenable to clip closure as long as sufficient pliable tissue surrounds the perforation site for effective anchoring of the clips (Video 9).

Coagulation grasping forceps

A monopolar grasping forceps (Coagrasper, Olympus Corp, Tokyo, Japan) dedicated for the coagulation of submucosal vessels during endoscopic mucosal resection (EMR) (**Fig. 9**) and endoscopic submucosal dissection (ESD) is available.[27] The device is designed for grasping, tenting, and sealing of readily accessible vessels, with suggested settings of 50 to 60 W, depending on the electrosurgical unit being used, using a soft coagulation mode. Although the device may also be suitable for other nonvariceal bleeding lesions, care regarding its use for the treatment of a VV in an ulcer is

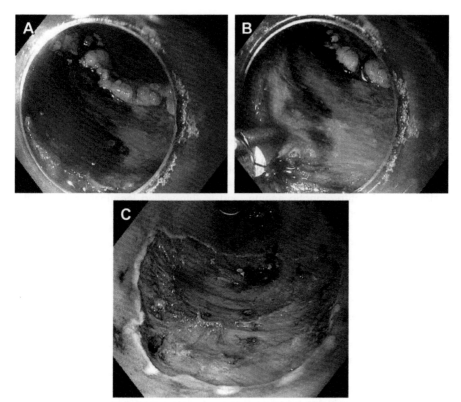

Fig. 9. (*A*) Active arterial bleeding during mucosal resection. (*B*) VV targeted using a coagulation grasping forceps. (*C*) Hemostasis secured.

warranted because grasping the vessel from an indurated base may result in vascular tearing and bleeding.

Argon plasma coagulation

Argon plasma coagulation (APC) is the preferred modality for the noncontact ablation of sporadic as well as diffuse angioectasias (see **Table 3**).[26,28] In situations when the lesions can be extensive (eg, gastric antral vascular ectasia [GAVE]), APC is more efficient and easier to use than contact thermal modalities. Although challenging at times, the APC probe should be fired at a distance of 1 to 3 mm from the target lesion. Antiperistaltic agents, such as glucagon and hyoscine, can be administered to decrease contractions and facilitate application of APC. Inadvertent probe-tissue contact during APC may result in localized pneumatosis, which is inconsequential; the use of ball-tipped APC probes may minimize this risk. The use of APC for radiation proctopathy necessitates full bowel cleansing because enema preparations are insufficient at clearing the colon of combustible gases. Overzealous APC of radiation-induced angioectasias should be avoided, as this can result in the formation of deep iatrogenic ulcers with poor healing in the setting of irradiated tissue (Video 10). The authors do not advocate the use of APC for larger-caliber vessels, as in peptic ulcers and gastric Dieulafoy lesions, because of the superficial nature of coagulation and heat sink effect from lack of compression of the vessel.

Mechanical Modalities

Through-the-scope clips

Several TTS mucosal clips are available, with differences in opening widths, rotation, and reopening capability (**Table 4**). There are no prospective trials that demonstrate the superiority of one type of TTS clip over another with regard to endoscopic hemostasis, and selection of a particular clip depends largely on device availability and operator preference.

TTS clips are suitable for sealing pliable vessels (<2 mm) and for closure of focal, nonindurated lesions or defects that are less than 2 cm in size. Clips are generally placed in a zipper fashion to seal the vessel or defect (Video 11). Unlike thermal modalities, clips are superficial and do not extend tissue injury.[29] Thus, when technically feasible, clips are preferred over thermal techniques in the setting of coagulopathy, use of antithrombotic agents, and in thin-walled locations, such as the cecum. As mentioned previously, clips are not appropriate for closure of deep, fibrotic ulcers and for targeting a vessel within an indurated base due to vascular avulsion and precipitation of potentially torrential bleeding (Video 12). Perforation from clip placement is exceedingly rare and is usually caused by operator error during blind, forceful advancement of the clipping device through an obscured field of view.

Over-the-scope clips

The OTSCs (Ovesco Endoscopy AG, Tübingen, Germany) are memory-shape nitinol clips that are akin to a bear claw trap. The clip comes preloaded in a bent state onto a cap, and its setup and deployment are analogous to a band ligation device. The Ovesco OTSCs are available in different diameters (11, 12, and 14 mm) and shapes of teeth. The nontraumatic (type A) clip with smooth, blunted teeth is used primarily for bleeding lesions in thin-walled segments of the gut, such as esophagus and colon, whereas the traumatic (type T) clip with sharper teeth may anchor better in firmer tissue and, thus, be more suitable for indurated lesions, such as peptic ulcers.[30] Suction is applied to engage the target lesion into the cap before clip release, which assumes its naturally closed state. It is important to center the bleeding point within the cap because some rolling of the lesion to the side may occur during suction. Once committed, suction should continuously be applied till clip deployment because the suction act will precipitate bleeding from the target vessel (Video 13). For indurated lesions, a dedicated tripronged anchoring device can assist in retracting the ulcer base into the cap. However, a certain amount of pliable tissue around the target vessel is still needed

Table 4 TTS clip devices				
Features	QuickClip2 (Olympus Corp)	QuickClipPro (Olympus Corp)	Resolution (Boston Scientific, Marlborough, MA)	Instinct (Cook Medical Inc, Bloomington, IN)
Opened jaw span (mm)	7 or 11	11	11	16
Rotation	Yes	Yes	Limited[a]	Yes
Reopening capability	No	Yes	Yes	Yes
Retention time (median)	2 wk	Not available	4 wk	Not available

[a] With sheath off.

to secure clip attachment regardless of what method is used to draw the targeted lesion into the cap.

The advantages of OTSCs relative to TTS clips include a greater compression force and volume of tissue captured between the prongs of the clip as well as improved access to certain lesions aided by the OTSC cap. Device limitations include the need to remove the endoscope for loading of the device and difficult passage through some areas, such as the cricopharyngeus or a diverticular-filled, angulated sigmoid colon. Mucosal lacerations and perforations as a result of passage of the device through narrowed lumens have been described.[31]

OTSC has been used for the treatment of various bleeding lesions, including Mallory-Weiss tears, peptic ulcers, Dieulafoy lesions, anastomotic ulcers, eroding tumors, and postpolypectomy ulcers, with success rates ranging from 71% to 100%.[30,32–36]

In some studies, an OTSC was used as salvage therapy for nonvariceal bleeding lesions that failed conventional hemostatic therapies, with success rates of 78% to 91%.[37,38] Cost-effectiveness studies comparing OTSCs versus TTS clips are awaited, although at the present time OTSCs can be used as potential salvage therapy or as a primary modality when placement of standard TTS clips is not deemed appropriate.

Band ligation

Although the most common application of EBL is for the prevention and treatment of esophageal variceal hemorrhage, it has also been used successfully for the management of a variety of nonvariceal bleeding lesions, including Mallory-Weiss tears, Dieulafoy lesions, arteriovenous malformations, postpolypectomy hemorrhage, and diverticular bleeding.[39,40]

Commercially available EBL kits fit onto diagnostic or therapeutic channel endoscopes. In the setting of active esophageal variceal bleeding, a therapeutic channel (3.7 mm) endoscope is preferable because of improved suction capability. Relative to rubber bands, neoprene bands have demonstrated early slippage in ex vivo studies because of their larger resting inner diameter and lower retraction force, although these findings have not been validated in clinical trials.[39] The authors' practice is to use a multiband ligator that enables up to 6 to 7 bands (depending on the brand used) to be placed in one session. The placement of greater than 6 bands per session was associated with significantly more total procedure times and misfired bands, without better patient outcomes, in one prospective trial.[41]

When active esophageal variceal bleeding is present, EBL should immediately target the bleeding site (Video 14). If the ligated varix is located at or near the gastroesophageal junction (GEJ), one can continue with banding of varices in a cephalad fashion, targeting varices in the distal 5 to 7 cm of the esophagus. If the initial banded site is in a higher location (eg, proximal or midesophagus), it is best to forego placement of additional bands distal to the index band, as the latter may become dislodged during endoscope passage, resulting in rebleeding (Video 15). For a more proximally situated varix with stigmata of recent bleeding (eg, nipple sign), EBL can start at the GEJ and conclude with the culprit varix. At least 2 bands should be available when targeting the offending varix to salvage for any potential misfiring of the initial band. In the setting of torrential hemorrhage, the exact bleeding site may not be localized. In this situation, initiation of EBL at the cardia or GEJ often allows variceal decompression and reduction in flow rate so that the actual bleeding site can be identified and ligated. One important technical aspect of successful banding is to capture enough of the varix into the band ligation cap. Limited, back-and-forth motion of the shaft of the endoscope while continuously applying suction often facilitates variceal entrapment into the cap and a red out of the field of view. The band will most likely slip off if sufficient tissue is not captured in the cap.

Potential adverse events following EBL for esophageal variceal bleeding include chest pain, postband ulcer bleeding, stricture formation, and perforation. Fortunately, the incidence of serious adverse events is very low. Chest pain is common after elective EBL, and a GI cocktail consisting of viscous lidocaine and liquid antacid should be prescribed after the procedure. The use of latex rubber bands probably should be avoided in patients who are allergic to latex, although no cases of serious allergic reactions have been reported to date.

EBL can be considered for the treatment of focal and nonfibrotic nonvariceal bleeding lesions that are less than 2 cm in size. Tangential lesions, such as a bleeding Mallory-Weiss tear along the cardia, may be more conducive to cap-assisted EBL than clip closure or thermal therapy. In the colon, EBL can be especially useful for ligation of stigmata of diverticular bleeding[42] that may otherwise be difficult to access by other endoscopic means, such as clips or thermal probes (**Fig. 10**). A tattoo or, preferably, a clip should be placed adjacent to the bleeding diverticulum to serve as a visual aid on reinsertion of the EBL-fitted endoscope (Video 16). The amount of suction used in this location is less, based on speculative concerns for creating delayed necrotic perforations.

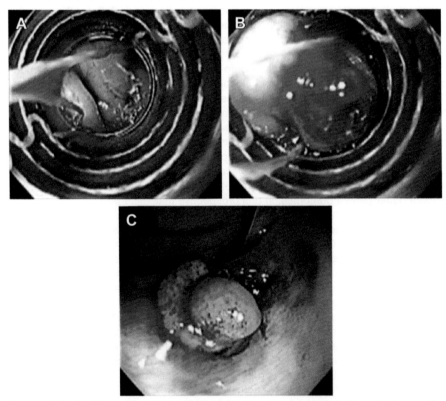

Fig. 10. (*A*) Bleeding colonic diverticulum. (*B*) Eversion of diverticulum during suction through the band ligation cap revealing visible vessel. (*C*) Post–band ligation appearance of treated diverticulum.

Detachable snares

Placement of a detachable nylon snare or endoloop (PolyLoop, Olympus Corp, Tokyo, Japan) is used primarily to prevent or treat bleeding during resection of large pedunculated polyps with thick stalks. However, encircling the stalk of a pedunculated polyp with a large head using the floppy endoloop device can be technically challenging, particularly if the working space is confined. Once constrained, the endoloop cannot be reopened and can become entangled inadvertently in the polyp head, rendering subsequent attempts at hot snare resection difficult or impossible. Thus, the authors prefer endoloop placement *after* polyp transection as long as a stump of sufficient length remains. Although the use of detachable stainless steel or nylon snares for ligation of gastric varices has been described,[43] the authors do not recommend this technique for fundal variceal hemorrhage because of endoloop slippage or difficulty ensaring fundal varices in a retroflexed position and the potential for a large ligation-induced ulcer that may result in life-threatening hemorrhage.

Endoscopic suturing

An endoscopic suturing system (OverStitch, Apollo Endosurgery, Austin, TX) is currently available on the market. It is affixed onto a specific double-channel endoscope (GIF 2T160 or GIF-2TH180, Olympus Corp, Tokyo, Japan) and consists of a curved needle with a detachable tip that carries an absorbable or nonabsorbable suture. The handle portion of the system is attached to the entrance port of the working channel, which activates transfer of the needle tip to enable passage and exit of the suture through tissue. A corkscrewlike retracting device (Helix, Apollo Endosurgery, Austin, TX) or a grasping forceps can be inserted through the second working channel of the endoscope to facilitate tissue retraction for suture placement. Stitches can be placed in an interrupted or running fashion without the need for device removal. A cinching catheter is used to tighten and release the suture.

Although endoscopic oversewing of a bleeding lesion is appealing, the need for a specialized endoscope and restricted maneuverability or access at certain locations of the gut will limit the use of this suturing system in the acute setting. However, the device seems suitable for the management of chronic bleeding caused by recalcitrant anastomotic ulcers[44] and for the prevention of delayed bleeding following EMR and ESD (**Fig. 11**).[45]

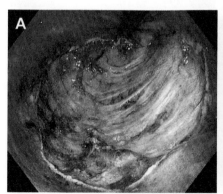
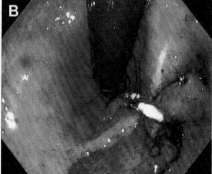

Fig. 11. (*A*) Large ESD defect with visualization of submucosal vessels. (*B*) Endoscopic suture closure of defect for prevention of delayed adverse events.

Cryotherapy

Cryotherapy results in superficial mucosal necrosis and ulceration, followed by re-epithelialization over several weeks.[46] Commercially available, catheter-based endoscopic cryotherapy systems use either liquid nitrogen (CSA Medical Inc, Lutherville, MD) or compressed carbon dioxide (CO_2) gas (Polar Wand, GI Supply, Camp Hill, PA) as cryogens. The clinical experience regarding the use of cryotherapy for endoscopic hemostasis is currently limited to the low-cost, portable CO_2 unit. A dedicated spray catheter is extended 1 to 2 cm distal to the tip of the endoscope, and a foot pedal activates the spraying of the compressed CO_2 cryogen. Drawbacks of cryotherapy include a cloudy field of view and delivery of a high volume of CO_2 gas (~8 L/min) during the procedure. Consequently, venting of the stomach necessitates either a dedicated decompression tube or a gastric length overtube, with constant monitoring of the abdomen for distention. The cryogenic spray is applied to the targeted mucosal surface until whitening (icing) occurs. This whitening is followed by thawing on termination of spraying. The freeze-thaw cycle is typically repeated 3 to 5 times per treatment session.

Cryotherapy has been applied with some success in the treatment of GAVE and radiation proctopathy.[47,48] The advantages of cryotherapy include the ease of use and ability to rapidly treat a large surface area. This modality seems suitable for ablation of mucosal vascular lesions, such as GAVE and radiation-induced telangiectasia, particularly when the distribution of these lesions is diffuse and extensive (**Fig. 12**). However, multiple treatment sessions seem necessary before a sustained response

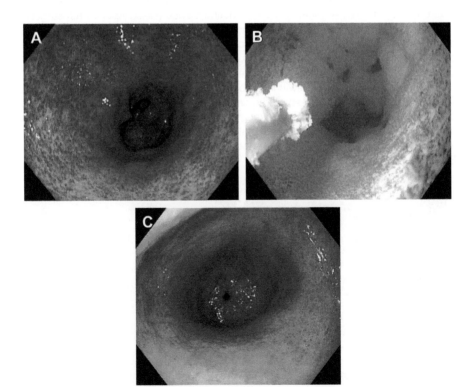

Fig. 12. (A) Diffuse and extensive GAVE. (B) Cryotherapy applied to affected mucosa. (C) Improved endoscopic appearance of GAVE at 1-month follow-up.

is achieved. The optimal treatment protocol based on the type of cryogen used, number of freeze-thaw cycles, duration of cryospray, and time interval between treatment sessions has not been determined.

Hemostatic Sprays

Hemostatic agents in the form of granules and powders are integrated in the military's first-aid kits for treatment of external bleeding from battlefield injuries.[49] TC-325 is a proprietary inorganic absorbent powder that forms an adherent coagulum at the targeted site. This agent has been incorporated into a handheld, CO_2 gas-propelled, push-button device for endoscopic hemostasis (Hemospray, Cook Medical Inc, Bloomington, IN).[50] The use of hemostatic sprays is limited to lesions or surface areas that are actively bleeding. Hemospray is commercially available in several countries, but is not yet approved by the Food and Drug Administration (FDA) for use in the United States.

The main appeal for Hemospray is its ease of use.[23] The spray can be delivered without precision to poorly accessible regions, such as the proximal lesser curve of the stomach and posterior wall of the duodenum, and temporize bleeding until a second-look endoscopy is performed. The coagulum sloughs off within a few days and is naturally excreted. Although endoscopic visualization is impaired during Hemospray application, the therapeutic benefit remains because precise targeting is not required. However, the delivery of subsequent therapies, should bleeding persist, is hindered by the cloudy field of view and adherent coagulum. It has been used to treat

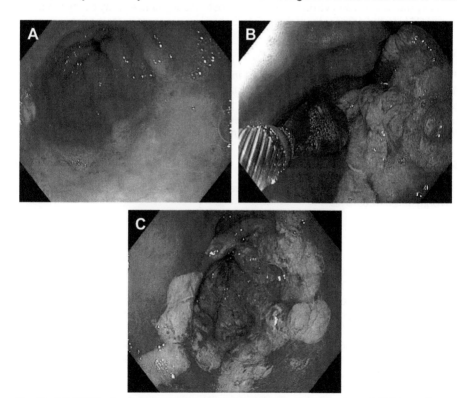

Fig. 13. (*A*) GAVE refractory to APC therapy. (*B*) Ablation of GAVE using a TTS RFA catheter. (*C*) Appearance of treated mucosa following RFA therapy.

a variety of nonvariceal bleeding lesions, including peptic ulcers (Video 17), esophageal ulcers, Dieulafoy lesions, postmucosectomy sites, and GAVE, with an overall success rate of 85% for sustained hemostasis.[51,52] Its use for tumor bleeding is marginally successful, an often difficult condition to treat endoscopically.[53,54] The reported adverse events are primarily technical in nature, including occlusion of the spray catheter or instrument channel.[52] Theoretic risks include inhalation of the powder when used in the esophagus in the absence of airway protection and intestinal obstruction from cast formation, although none of these potential adverse events have been reported to date. Despite the potential risk for venous embolization because the agent is delivered under pressure, Hemospray seems to be safe and effective at temporarily stopping variceal bleeding.[55] Additional data are needed, however, to further assess its efficacy and safety in the setting of variceal hemorrhage.

Miscellaneous Modalities

Dedicated stents for esophageal variceal tamponade have been developed as a more appealing alternative to balloon tamponade,[56] although these are not yet FDA approved for use in the United States. Certain lesions, such as postsphincterotomy bleeding and hemorrhage at cyst-gastrostomy sites, often respond favorably to placement of covered self-expandable metal stents and, thus, should be considered when conventional endoscopic therapies have failed.[57–59] The advent of a TTS radiofrequency ablation (RFA) catheter may render RFA more user friendly for ablation of GAVE (**Fig. 13**), although cost may prohibit RFA as the initial therapy for GAVE and for other mucosal-based vascular lesions.[60] Cost-efficacy studies may clarify the position of RFA as the primary therapy for GAVE or as rescue therapy for refractory cases.

SUMMARY

The endoscopist possesses an armamentarium of hemostatic devices and techniques for the management of acute GI bleeding. In addition to carefully evaluating the suitability of particular lesions for endoscopic hemostasis, the proper selection of tools and methods of use are among the key determinants for minimizing the risk of adverse events and for a successful endoscopic outcome.

SUPPLEMENTARY DATA

Supplementary data related to this article can be found online at http://dx.doi.org/10.1016/j.giec.2014.09.012.

REFERENCES

1. Laine L, Yang H, Chang SC, et al. Trends for incidence of hospitalization and death due to GI complications in the United States from 2001 to 2009. Am J Gastroenterol 2012;107:1190–5.
2. Hearnshaw SA, Logan RF, Lowe D, et al. Acute upper gastrointestinal bleeding in the UK: patient characteristics, diagnoses and outcomes in the 2007 UK audit. Gut 2011;60:1327–35.
3. Marmo R, Rotondano G, Piscopo R, et al. Dual therapy versus monotherapy in the endoscopic treatment of high-risk bleeding ulcers: a meta-analysis of controlled trials. Am J Gastroenterol 2007;102:279–89 [quiz: 469].
4. Barkun AN, Bardou M, Kuipers EJ, et al. International consensus recommendations on the management of patients with nonvariceal upper gastrointestinal bleeding. Ann Intern Med 2010;152:101–13.

5. Lin HJ, Hsieh YH, Tseng GY, et al. A prospective, randomized trial of large- versus small-volume endoscopic injection of epinephrine for peptic ulcer bleeding. Gastrointest Endosc 2002;55:615–9.

6. Croffie J, Somogyi L, Chuttani R, et al. Sclerosing agents for use in GI endoscopy. Gastrointest Endosc 2007;66:1–6.

7. Spier BJ, Fayyad AA, Lucey MR, et al. Bleeding stomal varices: case series and systematic review of the literature. Clin Gastroenterol Hepatol 2008;6:346–52.

8. Waring JP, Sanowski RA, Pardy K, et al. Does the addition of methylene blue to the sclerosant improve the accuracy of injections during variceal sclerotherapy? Gastrointest Endosc 1991;37:159–60.

9. Park WG, Yeh RW, Triadafilopoulos G. Injection therapies for variceal bleeding disorders of the GI tract. Gastrointest Endosc 2008;67:313–23.

10. ASGE Technology Committee, Bhat YM, Banerjee S, et al. Tissue adhesives: cyanoacrylate glue and fibrin sealant. Gastrointest Endosc 2013;78:209–15.

11. Cameron R, Binmoeller KF. Cyanoacrylate applications in the GI tract. Gastrointest Endosc 2013;77:846–57.

12. Seewald S, Ang TL, Imazu H, et al. A standardized injection technique and regimen ensures success and safety of N-butyl-2-cyanoacrylate injection for the treatment of gastric fundal varices (with videos). Gastrointest Endosc 2008;68:447–54.

13. Nguyen AJ, Baron TH, Burgart LJ, et al. 2-Octyl-cyanoacrylate (Dermabond), a new glue for variceal injection therapy: results of a preliminary animal study. Gastrointest Endosc 2002;55:572–5.

14. Rengstorff DS, Binmoeller KF. A pilot study of 2-octyl cyanoacrylate injection for treatment of gastric fundal varices in humans. Gastrointest Endosc 2004;59:553–8.

15. Reddy J, Wongkeesong LM, Buttar N, et al. Endoscopic injection of 2-ocytl cyanoacrylate (Dermabond) for the treatment of bleeding gastric varices [abstract]. Am J Gastroenterol 2005;100(Suppl 9):S363.

16. Sarin SK, Jain AK, Jain M, et al. A randomized controlled trial of cyanoacrylate versus alcohol injection in patients with isolated fundic varices. Am J Gastroenterol 2002;97:1010–5.

17. Tan PC, Hou MC, Lin HC, et al. A randomized trial of endoscopic treatment of acute gastric variceal hemorrhage: N-butyl-2-cyanoacrylate injection versus band ligation. Hepatology 2006;43:690–7.

18. Procaccini NJ, Al-Osaimi AM, Northup P, et al. Endoscopic cyanoacrylate versus transjugular intrahepatic portosystemic shunt for gastric variceal bleeding: a single-center U.S. analysis. Gastrointest Endosc 2009;70:881–7.

19. Cheng LF, Wang ZQ, Li CZ, et al. Low incidence of complications from endoscopic gastric variceal obturation with butyl cyanoacrylate. Clin Gastroenterol Hepatol 2010;8:760–6.

20. Romero-Castro R, Ellrichmann M, Ortiz-Moyano C, et al. EUS-guided coil versus cyanoacrylate therapy for the treatment of gastric varices: a multicenter study (with videos). Gastrointest Endosc 2013;78:711–21.

21. Wong Kee Song LM. Management of gastric varices. Clin Liver Dis 2012;1:158–62.

22. Levy MJ, Wong Kee Song LM. EUS-guided angiotherapy for gastric varices: coil, glue, and sticky issues. Gastrointest Endosc 2013;78:722–5.

23. ASGE Technology Committee, Wong Kee Song LM, Banerjee S, et al. Emerging technologies for endoscopic hemostasis. Gastrointest Endosc 2012;75:933–7.

24. Rao AS, Misra S, Buttar NS, et al. Combined endoscopic-interventional radiologic approach for the treatment of bleeding gastric varices in the setting of a large splenorenal shunt. Gastrointest Endosc 2012;76:1064–5.

25. Irani S, Kowdley K, Kozarek R. Gastric varices: an updated review of management. J Clin Gastroenterol 2011;45:133–48.
26. Morris ML, Tucker RD, Baron TH, et al. Electrosurgery in gastrointestinal endoscopy: principles to practice. Am J Gastroenterol 2009;104:1563–74.
27. Oyama T. Esophageal ESD: technique and prevention of complications. Gastrointest Endosc Clin N Am 2014;24:201–12.
28. Wong Kee Song LM, Baron TH. Endoscopic management of acute lower gastrointestinal bleeding. Am J Gastroenterol 2008;103:1881–7.
29. Anastassiades CP, Baron TH, Wong Kee Song LM. Endoscopic clipping for the management of gastrointestinal bleeding. Nat Clin Pract Gastroenterol Hepatol 2008;5:559–68.
30. Baron TH, Wong Kee Song LM, Ross A, et al. Use of an over-the-scope clipping device: multicenter retrospective results of the first U.S. experience (with videos). Gastrointest Endosc 2012;76:202–8.
31. Voermans RP, Le Moine O, von Renteln D, et al. Efficacy of endoscopic closure of acute perforations of the gastrointestinal tract. Clin Gastroenterol Hepatol 2012; 10:603–8.
32. Kirschniak A, Kratt T, Stüker D, et al. A new endoscopic over-the-scope clip system for treatment of lesions and bleeding in the GI tract: first clinical experiences. Gastrointest Endosc 2007;66:162–7.
33. Kirschniak A, Subotova N, Zieker D, et al. The over-the-scope clip (OTSC) for the treatment of gastrointestinal bleeding, perforations, and fistulas. Surg Endosc 2011;25:2901–5.
34. Albert JG, Friedrich-Rust M, Woeste G, et al. Benefit of a clipping device in use in intestinal bleeding and intestinal leakage. Gastrointest Endosc 2011;74:389–97.
35. Singhal S, Changela K, Papafragkakis H, et al. Over the scope clip: technique and expanding clinical applications. J Clin Gastroenterol 2013;47:749–56.
36. Alcaide N, Peñas-Herrero I, Sancho-Del-Val L, et al. Ovesco system for treatment of postpolypectomy bleeding after failure of conventional treatment. Rev Esp Enferm Dig 2014;106:55–8.
37. Manta R, Galloro G, Mangiavillano B, et al. Over-the-scope clip (OTSC) represents an effective endoscopic treatment for acute GI bleeding after failure of conventional techniques. Surg Endosc 2013;27:3162–4.
38. Chan SM, Chiu PW, Teoh AY, et al. Use of the over-the-scope clip for treatment of refractory upper gastrointestinal bleeding: a case series. Endoscopy 2014;46: 428–31.
39. Baron TH, Wong Kee Song LM. Endoscopic variceal band ligation. Am J Gastroenterol 2009;104:1083–5.
40. ASGE Technology Committee, Liu J, Petersen BT, et al. Endoscopic banding devices. Gastrointest Endosc 2008;68:217–21.
41. Ramirez FC, Colon VJ, Landan D, et al. The effects of the number of rubber bands placed at each endoscopic session upon variceal outcomes: a prospective, randomized study. Am J Gastroenterol 2007;102:1372–6.
42. Ishii N, Setoyama T, Deshpande GA, et al. Endoscopic band ligation for colonic diverticular hemorrhage. Gastrointest Endosc 2012;75:382–7.
43. Lee MS, Cho JY, Cheon YK, et al. Use of detachable snares and elastic bands for endoscopic control of bleeding from large gastric varices. Gastrointest Endosc 2002;56:83–8.
44. Jirapinyo P, Watson RR, Thompson CC. Use of a novel endoscopic suturing device to treat recalcitrant marginal ulceration (with video). Gastrointest Endosc 2012;76:435–9.

45. Kantsevoy SV, Bitner M, Mitrakov AA, et al. Endoscopic suturing closure of large mucosal defects after endoscopic submucosal dissection is technically feasible, fast, and eliminates the need for hospitalization (with videos). Gastrointest Endosc 2014;79:503-7.
46. Kantsevoy SV, Cruz-Correa MR, Vaughn CA, et al. Endoscopic cryotherapy for the treatment of bleeding mucosal vascular lesions of the GI tract: a pilot study. Gastrointest Endosc 2003;57:403-6.
47. Cho S, Zanati S, Yong E, et al. Endoscopic cryotherapy for the management of gastric antral vascular ectasia. Gastrointest Endosc 2008;68:895-902.
48. Moawad FJ, Maydonovitch CL, Horwhat JD. Efficacy of cryospray ablation for the treatment of chronic radiation proctitis in a pilot study. Dig Endosc 2013;25:174-9.
49. Gordy SD, Rhee P, Schreiber MA. Military applications of novel hemostatic devices. Expert Rev Med Devices 2011;8:41-7.
50. Barkun AN, Moosavi S, Martel M. Topical hemostatic agents: a systematic review with particular emphasis on endoscopic application in GI bleeding. Gastrointest Endosc 2013;7:692-700.
51. Sung JJ, Luo D, Wu JC, et al. Early clinical experience of the safety and effectiveness of Hemospray in achieving hemostasis in patients with acute peptic ulcer bleeding. Endoscopy 2011;43:291-5.
52. Morris AJ, Smith LA, Stanley A, et al. Hemospray for non-variceal upper gastrointestinal bleeding: results of the SEAL dataset (survey to evaluate the application of Hemospray in the luminal tract) [abstract]. Gastrointest Endosc 2012;75:AB133-4.
53. Chen YI, Barkun AN, Soulellis C, et al. Use of the endoscopically applied hemostatic powder TC-325 in cancer-related upper GI hemorrhage: preliminary experience (with video). Gastrointest Endosc 2012;75:1278-81.
54. Leblanc S, Vienne A, Dhooge M, et al. Early experience with a novel hemostatic powder used to treat upper GI bleeding related to malignancies or after therapeutic interventions. Gastrointest Endosc 2013;78:169-74.
55. Ibrahim M, El-Mikkawy A, Mostafa I, et al. Endoscopic treatment of acute variceal hemorrhage by using hemostatic powder TC-325: a prospective pilot study. Gastrointest Endosc 2013;78:769-73.
56. Wright G, Lewis H, Hogan B, et al. A self-expanding metal stent for complicated variceal hemorrhage: experience at a single center. Gastrointest Endosc 2010;71:71-8.
57. Itoi T, Yasuda I, Doi S, et al. Endoscopic hemostasis using covered metallic stent placement for uncontrolled post-endoscopic sphincterotomy bleeding. Endoscopy 2011;43:369-72.
58. Săftoiu A, Ciobanu L, Seicean A, et al. Arterial bleeding during EUS-guided pseudocyst drainage stopped by placement of a covered self-expandable metal stent. BMC Gastroenterol 2013;13:93.
59. Iwashita T, Lee JG, Nakai Y, et al. Successful management of arterial bleeding complicating endoscopic ultrasound-guided cystogastrostomy using a covered metallic stent. Endoscopy 2012;44(Suppl 2 UCTN):E370-1.
60. McGorisk T, Krishnan K, Keefer L, et al. Radiofrequency ablation for refractory gastric antral vascular ectasia (with video). Gastrointest Endosc 2013;78:584-8.

Sedation-Related Complications in Gastrointestinal Endoscopy

John J. Vargo II, MD, MPH

KEYWORDS

- Cardiopulomonary unplanned events • Pulse oximetry • Capnography

KEY POINTS

- Gastrointestinal endoscopy when undertaken by trained personnel after the appropriate preprocedural evaluation and in the right setting is a safe experience.
- However, clinicians should not be complacent in their lexicon when it comes to improving the safety of patients through further advances in the science of sedation and the lifetime journey of learning undertaken by gastrointestinal endoscopists.
- Significant challenges still exist in further quantifying the sedation risks to patients, optimizing physiologic monitoring, and sublimating the pharmacoeconomic and regulatory embroglios that limit the scope of practice and the quality of service delivered to patients.

"The real voyage of discovery consists not in seeking new landscapes, but in having new eyes."

—Marcel Proust

INTRODUCTION

Defining the risk of procedural sedation for gastrointestinal endoscopic procedures remains a vexing challenge. The definitions as to what constitutes a cardiopulmonary unplanned event (CUE) are beginning to take focus but the existing literature is an amalgam of various definitions and subjective outcomes, which provides a challenge to patient, practitioner, and researcher. The incidence of CUEs associated with gastrointestinal endoscopy is low. The rate of CUEs varies in the literature from 1 in 170 to 1 in 10,000.[1–3]

QUANTIFYING RISK OF SEDATION-RELATED UNPLANNED EVENTS

Early survey studies, such as that by Arrowsmith and colleagues,[4] culled data from more than 21,011 procedures and found the risks for serious unplanned events and death to be 5.4 and 0.3 per 1000 procedures, respectively. The most commonly

Department of Gastroenterology and Hepatology, Digestive Disease Institute, Cleveland Clinic, 9500 Euclid Avenue Desk A30, Cleveland, OH 44195, USA
E-mail address: vargoj@ccf.org

Gastrointest Endoscopy Clin N Am 25 (2015) 147–158
http://dx.doi.org/10.1016/j.giec.2014.09.009
1052-5157/15/$ – see front matter © 2015 Elsevier Inc. All rights reserved.

reported unplanned events were CUEs, which made up 40% of the reported events. By the very nature of its survey design, issues regarding ascertainment and recall bias could work in concert to underestimate the incidence of CUEs. Ganji and colleagues[5] used the outcomes data from a large hospital system in a case-control fashion to ascertain cardiovascular complications associated with endoscopic procedures. In this study, CUEs were defined as hypotension, chest pain or anginal equivalent, arrhythmia, or myocardial infarction occurring within 24 hours of endoscopy. Subjects were considered at risk for CUEs based on cardiac enzyme determinations, charges for cardiovascular medicines, and intensive care unit admission on the day of or after endoscopy. The rate of CUEs was 308 per 100,000 procedures. Independent CUE risk factors included male gender, the use of propofol, and the modified Goldman score.

Perhaps the best studies laying the framework for the incidence and risk factors for CUEs are by Sharma and colleagues[6] and Enestvedt and colleagues[7] analyzing the Clinical Outcomes Research Initiative endoscopic database. This database garners information from a total of 74 sites in the United States including academic, community, Veterans Affairs, and health maintenance organizations. In the work by Sharma and colleagues, data on 324,737 unique procedures including upper endoscopy, colonoscopy, endoscopic retrograde cholangiopancreatography (ERCP), and endoscopic ultrasound (EUS) using moderate sedation were reviewed. Overall, CUEs were reported in 0.9% of the procedures. Risk factors for these events included patient age, ascending American Society of Anesthesiologists (ASA) physical classification, inpatient procedures, nonuniversity sites and Veterans Affairs medical centers, the use of supplemental oxygen, and involvement of a trainee. Using the same database but with 1,590,648 unique endoscopic procedures, Enestvedt and colleagues found that an immediate adverse event occurred in 0.35% of all endoscopic procedures. Again, an increasing ASA physical classification was associated with a higher prevalence and was proportionally highest in ERCPs. In this study, however, the procedure-associated adverse event was defined as the rate of any immediate adverse event that prompted an unplanned intervention. This could include other unplanned events that were not cardiopulmonary in cause. Of the 470 serious adverse events, 14.5% of these included cardiopulmonary resuscitation. Risk factors for CUEs based on a review of the literature are listed in **Box 1**.

Box 1
Risk factors for cardiopulmonary unplanned events based on literature review

Age

ASA physical classification

Type of anesthesia

Inpatient

Setting (nonuniversity, Veterans Affairs)

Supplemental oxygen

Trainee involvement

Pulmonary disease

Cardiac disease

Obesity

A UNIVERSAL LEXICON FOR CARDIOPULMONARY UNPLANNED EVENTS

One of the challenges in this genre is the lack of standardized lexicon with a supporting attribution scheme and severity scale for CUEs. In 2009, a lexicon for endoscopic adverse events workshop was held.[8,9] The goals of this workshop were to provide clear definitions for adverse events and define levels of severity including the minimum threshold at which an adverse event should be documented and thus be counted and reported. Additionally, an analysis of the main risk factors for adverse events was undertaken, and how to consider the attribution with delayed events. **Table 1** lists the CUEs that in most cases would stem from the sedation regimen used during the endoscopic procedure. For all CUEs it is important to attest the timing of the event with the procedure. Occasionally, these events can occur preprocedurally, during the procedure, or immediately thereafter. It is rare for a cardiopulmonary event to occur more than 6 hours after the endoscopic procedure. In addition, an attribution context should be developed to determine whether the CUE is definitely, probably, possibly, or unlikely related to the endoscopic procedure.

Three aspects of CUEs should be kept in mind. First, "minor" events, such as transient hypoxemia, may not be clinically significant in most contexts. However, the predictive value of even these minor events has yet to be rigorously tested in a prospective fashion or within the purview of a large database. For example, even a minor episode of hypoxemia in a patient receiving supplemental oxygen could indicate significant alveolar hypoventilation. Second, because more serious CUEs, such as an oxygen saturation value of less than 85%, are uncommon, extremely large and costly randomized controlled trials are necessary to detect differences in safety and effectiveness of monitoring devices and sedation regimens. Third, because serious CUEs are rare, there are no data to show a decreased risk for such events by using various physiologic monitoring devices or sedation regimens. Because most critical event analyses have found prolonged hypoxemia secondary to respiratory depression is the triggering event in most cases of morbidity and mortality, we use such events as hypoxemia, disordered respiration, and apnea as the surrogate markers for the risk of serious CUE occurrence.

Table 1
Cardiopulmonary unplanned events

Category	Event	Definition
Cardiovascular	Hypotension	Blood pressure <90/50 or a decrease in systolic pressure of 20% of baseline
	Hypertension	Blood pressure >190/30 or increase in systolic blood pressure >20%
	Dysrhythmia	
	Cardiopulmonary arrest	
	Myocardial infarction	
	Cerebral vascular event	
Pulmonary	Hypoxia	SaO_2 <85%
	Apnea/hypopnea	
	Laryngospasm	
	Bronchospasm	
	Pneumonia	
	Pneumonitis	

Adapted from Romagnuolo J, Cotton PB, Eisen G, et al. Identifying and reporting risk factors for adverse events in endoscopy. Part 1: Cardiopulmonary events. Gastrointest Endosc 2011;73:579–85.

The continuum of sedation put forth by the ASA sponsored Committee for Sedation and Analgesia by Non-Anesthesiologists provides a useful yet nonvalidated construct for the risks of CUEs as a function of the depth of sedation (**Table 2**).[10] A critical component in determining the level of targeted sedation is a thorough preprocedural assessment of the patient coupled with the type of procedure that is planned. In most patients with normal physiology moderate sedation and analgesia should be targeted. In this state the patient exhibits purposeful response to verbal or tactile stimulation. The airway and spontaneous respiration are unaffected and cardiovascular function is usually maintained. As one progresses into deep sedation and analgesia the level of responsiveness to stimuli becomes muted and intervention may be necessary for airway maintenance and spontaneous respirations. It should be emphasized that a purposeful response to stimulation does not mean a withdrawal response to noxious stimuli. In the state of general anesthesia, there is no response even to noxious stimuli. Support is usually necessary for maintaining a patent airway and ventilation. Cardiovascular support additionally may be necessary.

An important component of safety is that the endoscopy team must be able to rescue the patient from unintended deeper levels of sedation. This requires the timely recognition of adverse physiology and the ability to act in terms of airway support, pharmacologic management, and in extreme cases, management of a cardiopulmonary arrest. What is the incidence of unintended deeper sedation during gastroenterologist-directed sedation? Patel and colleagues[11] used the combination of benzodiazepines and opioids in a balanced cohort of 80 ASA class I and II patients undergoing a variety of endoscopic procedures including esophagogastroduodenoscopy, colonoscopy, EUS, and ERCP. Levels of sedation were assessed every 3 minutes using the Modified Observer's Assessment of Alertness and Sedation score. Deep sedation occurred in 68% of the patients. In all instances the interval of the deep sedation was brief. The procedures with the highest incidence of deep sedation were ERCP (35%) and EUS (29%). Multivariate analysis found that ERCP and EUS were the only independent predictors of deep sedation. Other variables, such as procedure duration, body mass index, and dose of medication, were not found to be predictive of achieving deep sedation. These data suggest that unintended levels of deep

Table 2
Continuum of depth of sedation: definition of general anesthesia and levels of sedation/analgesia

	Minimal Sedation/ Anxiolysis	Moderate Sedation/ Analgesia	Deep Sedation/ Analgesia	General Anesthesia
Responsiveness	Normal response to verbal stimulation	Purposeful[a] response to verbal or tactile stimulation	Purposeful[a] response following repeated or painful stimulation	Unarousable even with painful stimulus
Airway	Unaffected	No intervention required	Intervention may be required	Intervention often required
Spontaneous ventilation	Unaffected	Adequate	May be inadequate	Frequently inadequate
Cardiovascular function	Unaffected	Usually maintained	Usually maintained	May be impaired

[a] Reflects withdrawal from a painful stimulus is not considered a purposeful response.

sedation are not uncommon and that because of their brevity at least in the confines of this study did not result in CUEs.

Age seems to be an important predictor of adverse events particularly with colonoscopy. Warren and colleagues[12] conducted an analysis of more than 53,000 Medicare beneficiaries aged 66 to 95 years who underwent outpatient colonoscopy. These subjects were matched with beneficiaries who did not undergo colonoscopy. This was a claims analysis that included cardiovascular events and procedure-related complications, such as bleeding and perforation leading to hospitalization or an emergency department visit. The adjusted risk of an unplanned event per 1000 persons steadily increased as the age of the patient increased. Comorbidities, such as chronic obstructive pulmonary disease, atrial fibrillation, congestive heart failure, and a history of stroke, also amplified this risk. Similarly, a pooled analysis found that octogenarians exhibited a higher rate of CUEs at rates 1.6 times higher than in patients of a younger age.[13]

HEMODYNAMICS

Although there is insufficient evidence to show a decrease in serious unplanned events during procedural sedation, hemodynamic monitoring using an automated blood pressure monitoring platform is endorsed by the American Society for Gastrointestinal Endoscopy and the ASA Task Force on Sedation and Analgesia by Non-Anesthesiologists.[10,14] Because most agents used for procedural sedation carry with them side effects that can cause hemodynamic instability, it is believed that early recognition will result in early intervention. In a prospective study, Fisher and colleagues[15] evaluated 130 consecutive ERCPs performed on 100 patients with the focus being the occurrence of cardiopulmonary complications. The patients were dichotomized by age (group 1, ≥65 years; group 2, <65 years). Outcomes including new electrocardiogram changes, elevated cardiac troponin levels, and the incidence of abnormal hemodynamic responses including oxygen desaturation, hypotension, and hypertension were assessed. Changes in the electrocardiogram were noted in 24% of the group 1 patients and 9.3% of the group 2 patients. Post-ERCP troponin rises were seen in six older patients and in none of the younger group. Of note, ST segment changes were seen in only two of the six patients who exhibited an elevated troponin level. Risk factors included a longer duration of the ERCP and a history of congestive heart failure.

Typically the blood pressure device should be cycled every 5 minutes if the patient remains hemodynamically stable, but should be cycled much more frequently when hypotension or hypertension are encountered. Continuous electrocardiography should be considered in patients undergoing procedures where deep sedation or general anesthesia is targeted, in those patients where advanced cardiopulmonary disease is present, and in elderly patients.

HYPOXEMIA, PULSE OXIMETRY, AND SUPPLEMENTAL OXYGEN

Transient mild hypoxemia is not uncommon and is probably inconsequential. It is encountered with sedated and unsedated procedures.[16] However, extended intervals of hypoxemia are associated with tachycardia[16,17] and coronary ischemia.[15,18–20] Supplemental oxygen can decrease the incidence of hypoxemia during sedated endoscopy[16,21] and has also been shown to reduce the incidence of ST segment depression in patients who have ischemic heart disease.[22] Despite universal recommendations for the use of pulse oximetry during endoscopic procedures, there are no data to suggest that its use decreases the incidence of significant CUEs. A systematic review of randomized controlled trials using perioperative pulse oximetry found no difference with regard to duration of hospital stay, postoperative complications, and mortality.[22] A recent meta-analysis and systematic review of pulse oximetry use in the perioperative period found that although the incidence of hypoxemia decreased 1.5 to 3 times when compared with patients without pulse oximetry monitoring, there was no effect on morbidity and mortality.[23] Despite the lack of data, the American Society for Gastrointestinal Endoscopy and the ASA recommend that pulse oximetry be used during endoscopic procedures and that supplemental oxygen is available.[10,14] This recommendation comes as a result of critical event analyses, which found that virtually all cardiopulmonary arrests are precipitated by unrecognized or undertreated prolonged intervals of hypoxemia.[24–27] It should be noted, however, that supplemental oxygen can mask alveolar hypoventilation and that there is a poor correlation between the clinical observation and objective measures of ventilation in the endoscopy suite.[28]

A potential source of measurement error known as signal averaging times can affect the degree of hypoxemia as shown in studies conducted in sleep laboratories.[29] This phenomenon has not been evaluated in endoscopy units. Additionally, manual recording of pulse oximetry values may lead to inaccurately elevated levels when compared with automated recording systems. This is likely because the personnel responsible for recording the physiologic data simply cannot keep up with the dynamic changes during sedated procedures.[30]

To clarify the risk factors of hypoxemia, Qadeer and colleagues[31] studied 123 patients undergoing a variety of endoscopic procedures using gastroenterologist-directed benzodiazepine and opioids. In this study hypoxemia was defined as an oxygen saturation of less than 90% for greater than or equal to 15 seconds. Overall there were a total of 132 hypoxemic events in 85 patients. A total of 85% of these events occurred within 5 minutes of the administration of the sedation agent or during endoscopic intubation. Only one-third of these events were associated with any abnormal ventilation pattern as seen with capnography. An independent risk factor for hypoxemia was the development of abnormal ventilation or apnea. Of note is that the ASA physical classification was limited to grades 1 through 3, and that an ascending ASA score was not a risk factor for apnea. Other risk factors for hypoxemia include difficulty with esophageal intubation, a prolonged procedure, emergent indications for the endoscopic procedure, the presence of a significant comorbid illness, and a baseline oxygen level of less than 95%.[6,17,21] The risk factors for hypoxemia in the setting of propofol-mediated sedation were analyzed in a multicenter randomized study using capnographic monitoring. These included older age, elevated body mass index, history of sleep apnea, monitoring without capnography, and total dose of either propofol or ketamine.[32]

Can extended monitoring of respiratory activity augment the level of safety during gastrointestinal endoscopy? Transcutaneous carbon dioxide monitoring ($PtCO_2$) is a noninvasive method for measuring arterial carbon dioxide. Typically a heated electrode is placed on the skin, which allows the microcirculation to "arterialize." There is a diffusion of the carbon dioxide into an electrolyte solution, which produces carbonic acid. Using the Henderson-Hasselbach equation, a pH reading is obtained, which allows for a calculation of the arterial carbon dioxide level. Nelson and colleagues[28] randomized 395 patients undergoing ERCP to standard monitoring or standard monitoring coupled with $PtCO_2$ monitoring. In the standard monitoring group, significantly more patients exhibited CO_2 retention of greater than 40 mm Hg. Predictors for CO_2 retention included the combination of a benzodiazepine and opioid for sedation and analgesia, higher degree of oxygen desaturation, higher rates of supplemental oxygen delivery, the use of naloxone, and a higher baseline $PtCO_2$.

Capnography has also been used to obtain a graphic assessment of respiratory activity during endoscopic procedures. This is based on the principle that carbon dioxide absorbs light at 420 nm, which is in the infrared region of the electromagnetic spectrum. The carbon dioxide partial pressure can therefore be obtained throughout the respiratory cycle and the graphic representation of this mirrors the inspiratory and expiratory activity of the patient.[33] In a series of 49 patients undergoing prolonged endoscopic procedures using gastroenterologist-directed sedation, capnography was found to be more sensitive than pulse oximetry or direct observation of respiratory activity in the detection of apnea or disordered respiration.[34]

There have been four randomized controlled trials that have used capnography for endoscopic procedures (**Table 3**).[28,35–37] Lightdale and colleagues[35] randomized 163 pediatric patients undergoing upper endoscopy and colonoscopy or combination of both to standard monitoring with or without the addition of capnography. In the standard monitoring arm the capnography data were blinded to the procedure team. The primary aim of this study was to determine whether interventions based on capnography reduced the incidence of hypoxemia, with the sedation target being moderate sedation using the combination of a benzodiazepine and opioid. Subjects titrated with capnography data were significantly less likely to experience hypoxemia (11% vs 24%; $P<.03$). Qadeer and colleagues[36] randomized 247 patients undergoing gastroenterologist-directed sedation for ERCP and EUS to either standard monitoring or capnography in addition to standard monitoring. Hypoxemia developed in 69% of the patients in the standard sedation arm compared with only 46% in the capnography arm ($P<.001$). In subjects monitored with capnography, there was also a significantly decreased incidence of severe hypoxemia (SaO_2 <85%) and apnea. Beitz and colleagues[37] randomized 760 patients undergoing colonoscopy with gastroenterologist-directed propofol sedation. Again, the incidence of hypoxemia was lower in the capnography arm (38.9% vs 53.2%; $P<.001$), as was the incidence of severe hypoxemia ($SaO_2 \leq 85\%$; 3.7% vs 7.8%; $P = .018$). Friedrich-Rust and colleagues[32] randomized a total of 533 patients to standard monitoring alone or standard monitoring with capnography in patients sedated with propofol. In this study, the control arm did not have blinded capnography data. Additionally, propofol-mediated sedation was used for all procedures but included anesthesiologist-, gastroenterologist-, and nurse-administered propofol sedation. Assignment of the personnel administering propofol was stratified to eliminate potential confounding. The incidence of hypoxemia was significantly lower in patients titrated with capnography monitoring when compared with standard monitoring (18% vs 32%; $P = .0009$).

It is important to emphasize that there are currently no data available addressing the use of capnography monitoring for adult patients undergoing elective upper endoscopy or colonoscopy where moderate sedation is targeted. The ASA has issued an opinion regarding the use of capnography during moderate sedation stating "during moderate or deep sedation the adequacy of ventilation shall be evaluated by continual observation of qualitative clinical signs and monitoring for the presence of exhaled carbon dioxide unless precluded or invalidated by the nature of the patient or equipment."[38] Additionally, some authors point to the results of the ASA's closed claims analysis involving monitored anesthesia care cases and concludes that capnography should be used for instances of procedural sedation.[39]

Table 3
Summary of randomized, controlled trials using capnography

Author	Procedure Type	Number of Subjects	Sedation Type	Reduction in Hypoxemia	Reduction in Apnea	Reduction in Severe Hypoxemia
Lightdale et al,[35] 2006	Pediatric EGD or colonoscopy	163	GI-directed benzodiazepine/opioid	Yes	Not measured	Not measured
Qadeer et al,[36] 2009	ERCP or EUS	247	GI-directed benzodiazepine/opioid	Yes	Yes	Yes
Beitz et al,[37] 2012	Colonoscopy	760	GI-directed propofol	Yes	Not measured	Yes
Friedrich-Rust et al,[32] 2013	Colonoscopy ± EGD	553	Anesthesiologist-directed propofol; GI-directed sedation Nurse-directed sedation	Yes	Not measured	No

Abbreviations: EGD, esophagogastroduodenoscopy; GI, gastrointestinal.

DOES PROPOFOL EQUATE TO ENHANCED SAFETY?

Is propofol-mediated sedation the safest route for patients undergoing endoscopic procedures? Korman and colleagues[40] in a small observational study scrutinized the effect of propofol anesthesia on force application during colonoscopy. This was a multicenter study involving academic gastroenterology training programs and community ambulatory surgical centers. Significantly more axial and radial force was applied to the colonoscope in patients receiving propofol-mediated sedation when compared with those receiving moderate sedation with the combination of a benzodiazepine and opioid. Clearly this observation is provocative but far from definitive. However, when patients are in a state of deep sedation or general anesthesia they are unable to register reactions to increased tension or pressure placed on the mesentery or colonic wall. In a population-based study involving 35,128 procedures with anesthesia services, Cooper and colleagues[41] found that performing a colonoscopy with anesthesiologist-directed sedation was an independent risk factor for any increased complication risk (odds ratio, 1.46; 95% confidence interval, 1.09–1.94). In this study, complications included hospitalizations for splenic rupture or trauma, aspiration pneumonia, or colonic perforation within 30 days of the colonoscopy.

PSYCHOMOTOR RECOVERY

It is important to realize that the existing scoring systems for recovery following procedural sedation only address the recovery of baseline physiologic parameters and gross motor skills.[42] When can the patient safely resume the activities of daily living following an endoscopic procedure? Willey and colleagues[43] studied a battery of psychomotor tests in a cohort of 31 patients undergoing elective outpatient upper endoscopy targeting moderate sedation with meperidine and midazolam. The battery of tests included the letter cancellation test, multiple-choice reaction time, critical tracking test, and an assessment of manual dexterity. At the point in recovery where the patients achieved an Aldrete score of 10, all four psychomotor tests indicated a significant average decrease from baseline cognitive and motor function. Simultaneous use of the letter cancellation and multiple-choice reaction time tests were believed to be the best combination in assessing recovery of psychomotor function. Riphaus and colleagues[44] addressed the quality of psychomotor recovery after propofol sedation for routine endoscopy. A total of 100 patients undergoing routine upper or lower endoscopy were randomized to receive either propofol alone or the combination of midazolam and meperidine. Patients receiving propofol recovered their baseline driving skills via a simulator 2 hours postsedation. However, the time needed to complete the number connection test after sedation did not differ between the sedation arms suggesting that at least on this test, a degree of psychomotor recovery delay was present even for those receiving propofol. Horiuchi and colleagues[45,46] have also studied psychomotoric recovery following propofol-mediated sedation. The authors found baseline psychomotoric skills as assessed by a driving simulator had returned to baseline 1 hour following the procedure. In the study where colonoscopy was addressed, the number connection test additionally had returned to baseline 1 hour following the procedure. Why the difference between the Horiuchi and Riphaus studies? Potential explanations for this difference include the higher dose of propofol in the Riphuas study and perhaps unidentified pharmacokinetic differences in the study populations. At this point, given that some studies show a delay in psychomotoric recovery with propofol, a rapid return to baseline activities of daily living still cannot be recommended.

TRAINING: THE FINAL FRONTIER

To provide a universal educational platform for procedural sedation, a Multisociety Sedation Curriculum for Gastrointestinal Endoscopy was created to provide trainees and established practitioners alike a programmatic approach to achieve competency in procedural sedation.[47] With the development of online courses and high-fidelity simulation models, each member of the endoscopy team has the opportunity to maximize their skill set. The natural outgrowth of this is the early recognition and appropriate management of CUEs.

SUMMARY

Gastrointestinal endoscopy when undertaken by trained personnel after the appropriate preprocedural evaluation and in the right setting is a safe experience. However, clinicians should not be complacent in the lexicon when it comes to improving the safety of patients through further advances in the science of sedation and the lifetime journey of learning undertaken by gastrointestinal endoscopists. Significant challenges exist in further quantifying the sedation risks to patients, optimizing physiologic monitoring, and sublimating the pharmacoeconomic and regulatory embroglios that limit the scope of practice and the quality of the service delivered to patients.

REFERENCES

1. Silvis SE, Nebel O, Rogers G, et al. Endoscopic complications. Results of the 1974 American Society for Gastrointestinal Endoscopy Survey. JAMA 1976;235: 928–30.
2. Quine MA, Bell GD, McCloy RF, et al. Prospective audit of upper gastrointestinal endoscopy in two regions of England: safety staffing and sedation methods. Gut 1995;36:462–7.
3. Froelich F, Converse JJ, Fried M. Conscious sedation, clinically relevant complications and monitoring of endoscopy: results of a nationwide survey in Switzerland. Endoscopy 1994;26:231–4.
4. Arrowsmith JB, Gertsman BB, Fleischer DE, et al. Results from the American Society for Gastrointestinal Endoscopy/U.S. Food and Drug Administration collaborative study on complication rates and drug use during gastrointestinal endoscopy. Gastrointest Endosc 1991;37:421–7.
5. Ganji S, Saidia F, Patel K, et al. Cardiovascular complications after GI endoscopy: occurrence and risks in a large hospital system. Gastrointest Endosc 2004;60:679–85.
6. Sharma VK, Nguyen CC, Crowell MD, et al. A national study of cardiopulmonary unplanned events after GI endoscopy. Gastrointest Endosc 2007;66:27–33.
7. Enestvedt DK, Eisen GM, Holub J, et al. Is the American Society of Anesthesiologists classification useful in risk stratification for endoscopic procedures? Gastrointest Endosc 2013;77:464–71.
8. Cotton PB, Eisen GM, Aabakken L, et al. A lexicon for endoscopic adverse events: report of an ASGE Workshop. Gastrointest Endosc 2010;71:446–54.
9. Romagnuolo J, Cotton PB, Eisen G, et al. Identifying and reporting risk factors for adverse events in endoscopy. Part 1: Cardiopulmonary events. Gastrointest Endosc 2011;73:579–85.
10. Gross JB, Bailey PL, Connis RT, et al, American Society of Anesthesiologists Task force on Sedation and Analgesia by Non-Anesthesiologists. Practice guidelines for sedation and analgesia by non-anesthesiologists. Anesthesiology 2002;96: 1004–17.

11. Patel S, Vargo JJ, Khandwala F, et al. Deep sedation occurs frequently during elective endoscopy with material meperidine and midazolam am. Am J Gastroenterol 2005;100:2689–95.

12. Warren JL, Klabunde CN, Mariotto AB, et al. Adverse events after outpatient colonoscopy in the Medicare population. Ann Intern Med 2009;150:849–57.

13. Day LW, Kwon A, Inadomi JM, et al. Adverse events in older patients undergoing colonoscopy: a systematic review and meta-analysis. Gastrointest Endosc 2011; 74:885–96.

14. Waring JP, Baron TH, Hirota WK, et al. Guidelines for conscious sedation and monitoring during gastrointestinal endoscopy. Gastrointest Endosc 2003;58: 317–22.

15. Fisher L, Fisher A, Thomson A. Cardiopulmonary complications of ERCP in older patients. Gastrointest Endosc 2006;63:948–55.

16. Griffin SM, Chung SC, Leung JW, et al. Effect of intranasal oxygen on hypoxia and ancreatography. BMJ 1990;300:83–4.

17. Woods SD, Chung SC, Leung JW, et al. Hypoxemia and tachycardia during endoscopic retrograde cholangiopancreatography: detection by pulse oximetry. Gastrointest Endosc 1989;35:523–5.

18. Johnston ST, McKenna A, Tham TC. Silent myocardial ischemia during endoscopic retrograde cholangiopancreatography. Endoscopy 2003;35:1039–42.

19. Jarrell KR, O'Connor JW, Slack J, et al. Effect of supplemental oxygen on cardiopulmonary changes during gastrointestinal endoscopy. Gastrointest Endosc 1994;40:665–70.

20. Holm C, Christiansen M, Rasmussen V, et al. Hypoxemia and myocardial ischemia during colonoscopy. Scand J Gastroenterol 1998;33:769–72.

21. Bell GD, Bown S, Morden A. Prevention of hypoxemia during upper gastrointestinal endoscopy by means of oxygen via nasal cannulae. Lancet 1987;312: 1022–4.

22. Pedersen T, Moller AM, Pedersen BD. Pulse oximetry for perioperative monitoring: systematic review of randomized, controlled trials. Anesth Analg 2003; 96:426–31.

23. Pedersen T, Nicholson A, Hovhannisyan K, et al. Pulse oximetry for perioperative monitoring. Cochrane Database Syst Rev 2014;(3):CD002013. Accessed August 29, 2014. http://dx.doi.org/10.1002/14651858.CD002013.pub3.

24. Malviya S, Voepel-Lewis T, Tait AR. Adverse events and risk factors associated with sedation of children by non-anesthesiologists. Anesth Analg 1997;85: 1207–13.

25. Coté CJ, Notterman DA, Karl HW, et al. Adverse events and risk factors in pediatrics: a critical incident analysis of contributing factors. Pediatrics 2000;105:805–14.

26. Hutton P, Clutton-Brock T. The benefits and pitfalls of pulse oximetry. BMJ 1993; 307:457–8.

27. Davidson JA, Hosie HE. Limitations of pulse oximetry: respiratory insufficiency, a failure of detection. BMJ 1993;307:372–3.

28. Nelson DB, Freeman ML, Silvis ST, et al. A randomized controlled trial of transcutaneous carbon dioxide monitoring during ERCP. Gastrointest Endosc 2000;51: 288–95.

29. Zafar S, Ayappa I, Norman R, et al. Choice of oximeter affects apnea hypopnea index. Chest 2005;127:80–8.

30. Taenzor H, Pyke J, Eric MD, et al. A comparison of oxygen saturation data in patients with low oxygen saturation using automated continuous monitoring and intermittent manual data charting. Anesth Analg 2014;118:326–31.

31. Qadeer MA, Lopez AR, Dumot JA, et al. Hypoxemia during moderate sedation for gastrointestinal endoscopy: causes and associations. Digestion 2011;84:37–45.

32. Friedrich-Rust M, Welte M, Welte C, et al. Capnography monitoring of propofol basis sedation during colonoscopy. Endoscopy 2014;46:236–44.

33. Soto RG, Fu ES, Vila H, et al. Capnography accurately detects apnea during monitored anesthesia care. Anesth Analg 2004;99:379–82.

34. Zuccaro G, Radealli F, Vargo J, et al. Routine use of supplemental oxygen prevents recognition of prolonged apnea during endoscopy. Gastrointest Endosc 2000;51:AB141.

35. Lightdale JR, Goldmann DA, Feldman HA, et al. Medical history and capnography improves patient monitoring during moderate sedation: a randomized controlled trial. Pediatrics 2006;170:e1170–8.

36. Qadeer MA, Vargo JJ, Dumot JA, et al. Capnography monitoring of respiratory activity improves safety of sedation for endoscopic cholangiopancreatography and ultrasonography. Gastroenterology 2009;136:1568–76.

37. Beitz A, Riphaus A, Meining A, et al. Capnography monitoring reduces the incidence of arterial oxygen desaturation and hypoxemia during propofol sedation for colonoscopy: a randomized controlled study: (ColoCap Study). Am J Gastroenterol 2012;107:1205–12.

38. Available at: www.asahq.org/For-Members/Standards-Guidelines-and-Statements.aspx. Accessed August 31, 2014.

39. Bhananker SM, Posner KL, Cheney FW, et al. Injury and liability associated with monitored in Ossetia care: a closed claims analysis. Anesthesiology 2006;104:228–34.

40. Korman LY, Haddad NG, Metz DC, et al. Effect of propofol anesthesia on force application during colonoscopy. Gastrointest Endosc 2014;76:1–6.

41. Cooper GS, Kou TD, Rex DK. Complications following colonoscopy with anesthesia assistance. JAMA Intern Med 2013;173:551–6.

42. Aldrete JA, Kroulick D. A postanesthetic recovery score. Anesth Analg 1970;49:924–34.

43. Willey J, Vargo JJ, Connor JT, et al. Quantitative assessment of psychomotor recovery after sedation and analgesia for outpatient EGD. Gastrointest Endosc 2002;56:810–6.

44. Riphaus A, Gstettenbauer T, Frenz MD, et al. Quality of psychomotor recovery after propofol sedation for routine endoscopy: a randomized and controlled study. Endoscopy 2006;38:677–83.

45. Horiuchi A, Nakayama Y, Fujii H, et al. Psychomotor recovery and blood propofol level in colonoscopy when using propofol sedation. Gastrointest Endosc 2012;75:506–12.

46. Horiuchi A, Nakayama Y, Katayama Y, et al. Safety and driving ability following low-dose propofol sedation. Digestion 2008;78:190–4.

47. Vargo JJ, DeLegge MH, Feld AD, et al. Multisociety Sedation Curriculum for Gastrointestinal Endoscopy Task Force. Multisociety sedation curriculum for gastrointestinal endoscopy. Gastrointest Endosc 2012;76:e1–25.

New Devices and Techniques for Handling Adverse Events: Claw, Suture, or Cover?

Nikhil A. Kumta, MD, Christine Boumitri, MD,
Michel Kahaleh, MD, FASGE*

KEYWORDS

- Endoscopic closure • Endoscopic suturing • Over-the-scope-clip
- Cardiac septal defect occluder • Perforation • Fistula • Anastomotic leak

KEY POINTS

- Two devices are currently approved by the US Food and Drug Administration for endoscopic closure of gastrointestinal defects, including perforations, anastomotic leaks, and fistulas: the over-the-scope clip and the endoscopic suturing system.
- A third device, the cardiac septal defect occluder, has been adapted for use in the gastrointestinal tract.
- Devices are under development to facilitate closure by improving access to defects and simplifying closure.

INTRODUCTION

With the development of natural orifice translumenal endoscopic surgery (NOTES) and as therapeutic endoscopic procedures become more sophisticated, closure for iatrogenic mural defects of the gastrointestinal (GI) tract has become an evolving area in advanced interventional endoscopy.[1] Endoscopic clips were among the first endoscopic devices used for closure of perforations but are less effective for closure of larger defects, because of limited opening distance between jaws, low closure force, and inability to accomplish deep tissue capture.[2] Devices and techniques are under development to facilitate closure of GI wall defects. The ideal closure device should be inexpensive, safe, readily available (on demand), and easy to use and should provide rapid, reliable, and durable closure.[3]

INDICATIONS/CONTRAINDICATIONS

Endoscopic closure may be indicated in cases of inflammatory or neoplastic fistulas, dehiscence of surgical anastomoses, and iatrogenic or spontaneous perforations of

Division of Gastroenterology and Hepatology, Weill Cornell Medical College, 1305 York Avenue, 4th Floor, New York, NY 10021, USA
* Corresponding author.
E-mail address: MKahaleh@gmail.com

Gastrointest Endoscopy Clin N Am 25 (2015) 159–168
http://dx.doi.org/10.1016/j.giec.2014.09.011   giendo.theclinics.com

the GI tract.[3] Advanced endoscopic procedures, including large polypectomies, endoscopic mucosal resection (EMR), endoscopic submucosal dissection (ESD), and peroral endoscopic myotomy (POEM), have become more commonplace, and the mural defects caused by the procedures themselves are amenable to endoscopic closure. Complications from bariatric surgery and colorectal surgery, including chronic anastomotic leaks and marginal ulcers, may also benefit from endoscopic alternatives.[4] An important contraindication to isolated endoscopic closure involves the clinical setting of delayed perforation with peritonitis and septic fluid collections.[5] **Table 1** lists indications and contraindications for endoscopic closure.

DEVICES

In the mid 1990s, endoscopic closure of gastric and colonic perforations with hemostatic clips was reported.[2,6] Since then, a variety of techniques have been used to close mucosal defects caused by polypectomy, EMR, ESD, POEM, and electrocautery.[4] The need for endoscopic solutions for closure of intentional transmural defects has continued to increase, particularly with current NOTES driven efforts at full-thickness resection.[7,8] The techniques used in human subjects include an over-the-scope clip (OTSC) (OVESCO, Tübingen, Germany; Padlock, Aponos Medical, Kingston, NH), the endoscopic suturing system (OverStitch, Apollo Endosurgery, TX), and cardiac septal defect occluders.[3]

Over-the-Scope Clip

The OTSC system is an endoscopic hemostatic clip that was first intended for the treatment of nonvariceal GI bleeding.[9] These clips, also referred to as the "bear claw", are made of elastic biocompatible nitinol capable of full-thickness closure through tissue approximation.[9,10] The device was approved by the US Food and Drug Administration (FDA) in 2010.[3]

Compared with standard through-the-scope (TTS) clips, OTSCs can provide single application closure for defects up to 2 cm.[5] The OTSC is believed to produce more durable closure than standard TTS clips, because of its ability to apply a greater compressive force, and when used in conjunction with specially designed tissue graspers provides single-layer full-thickness closure of open defects.[10–12] The OTSC has also been used for resection of submucosal tumors, treatment of bleeding lesions, and esophageal stent fixation.[10]

Endoscopic Suturing System

The endoscopic suturing system is a disposable, single-use suturing device that allows placement of running or interrupted full-thickness sutures using either permanent (polypropylene) or absorbable suture material.[13] In contrast to hemostatic endoscopic clips, the device was specifically designed to simulate hand sewing for any type of

Table 1
Endoscopic closure: indications and contraindications

Indications	Contraindications
Fistulas (inflammatory or neoplastic)	Uncontained perforations
Dehiscence of surgical anastomosis	Peritonitis
Perforations (iatrogenic or spontaneous)	
Mural defects from large polypectomies, EMR, ESD, POEM	
Anastomotic leaks	
Marginal ulcers	

tissue approximation.[14] The device is mounted onto a double-channel therapeutic endoscope.[3,13] One of the advantages of the device is its ability to be reloaded as many times as needed without the endoscope being removed from the patient.[14] The suturing system has rapidly been adopted and used successfully to close persistent gastrocutaneous fistulas, esophageal fistulas, full-thickness resection sites in the stomach and colon, as well as perforations (**Fig. 1**). Other popular applications include anchoring esophageal stents to prevent migration, suture nonhealing ulcers, bariatric sleeve gastroplasty, revision of gastrojejunal anastomosis after Roux-en-Y gastric bypass, and closing large post-ESD defects.[14]

Cardiac Septal Defect Occluder

The Amplatzer Septal Occluder (ASO) (AGA Medical Group, MN) is a device that was developed for the occlusion of cardiac septal defects but has been used off label for the closure of fistulas in the GI tract.[3] The device consists of 2 self-expandable round disks made of nitinol wire mesh, which are linked together by a short connecting waist. A handful of case reports describe their use in closure of gastrocolonic and esophagotracheal fistulas.[15–19]

Other

Omental plug closure has been used for years and has been recently studied as a reliable method for closure of acute peptic ulcer perforations.[20,21] The omental plug is maintained in position within the lumen with mucosal clips. Other techniques that have been evaluated for endoscopic closure include trial of no closure of defect, self-approximating tunnel/flap, and gastropexy.[3] Devices in animal studies include bioabsorbable foam plugs, mucosal clips, Endoloops (Ethicon, NJ), flexible linear staplers, and circular staplers.[3,22,23]

EXPLANATION OF TECHNIQUE
Over-the-Scope Clip

This discussion focuses mainly on the OVESCO clip, which is the most commonly used OTSC. A clear cap holds a nitinol clip that is affixed to the tip of the endoscope (**Fig. 2**A, B). Caps are available in 3 diameters to accommodate the sizes of various endoscopes: 11 mm, 12 mm, and 14 mm.[3] Caps are also available in different depths to change the amount of tissue that can be grasped during approximation. A clip

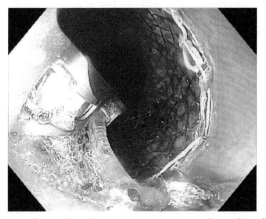

Fig. 1. Suture of an esophageal metal stent to cover an esophageal perforation.

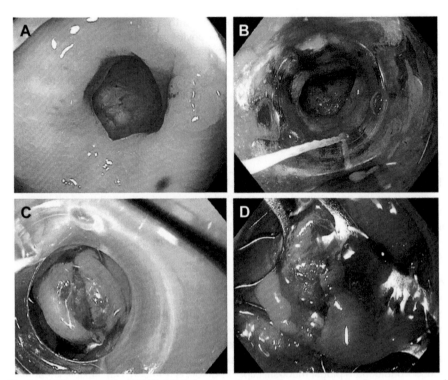

Fig. 2. OTSC closure of a POEM. (*A*) Colonic perforation from endoscope shown as mucosal defect with underlying fat. (*B*) Placement of OTSC endoscopic cap device over the mucosal defect. The metal clip can be seen through the clear endoscopic cap. (*C*) After deployment of the clip. The clip is entrapping the tissue, and the clip is no longer seen on the exterior of the endoscopic cap. (*D*) Relook endoscopy showing complete full-thickness closure of the mucosal defect.

release is incorporated into the cap. A thread is pulled retrograde through the working channel of the endoscope, where it is fixed onto a hand wheel at the working channel access port of the scope. Alternatively, the Padlock clip has a catheter that runs alongside the insertion tube of the endoscope and is attached to a syringelike trigger, which releases the radial compression clip (**Fig. 3**). The endoscope is then inserted to the desired target site of closure. Both OTSC devices can be deployed by using suction to bring the targeted areas into the cap.

Two devices exist to aid in tissue apposition and are inserted through the working channel. The first is a twin grasper that has a unique capability to open left-sided and right-sided graspers to obtain opposite sides of an open defect and appose the tissue, theoretically in a full-thickness single-layer-type closure. The tissue in the graspers can then be pulled into the cap device in preparation for deployment. The second device is a retractable tissue anchor set (3 curved nitinol needles), which is also used for approximation of the tissue.

During clip application, the tissue is either suctioned into the cap to secure the tissue or the tissue graspers are more ideally used to pull the captured tissue into the cap for a more robust and deeper tissue capture. Suction can also be used to supplement this capture method. Turning the hand wheel attached to the working channel near the hand dials subsequently results in deployment of the clip by compressing the entrapped tissue.[10] The OTSC can be conveniently used in suitably sized (<2 cm) colonic

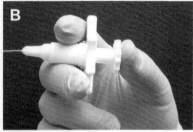
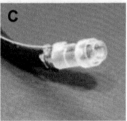

Fig. 3. (*A*) Padlock OTSC and (*B*) deployment catheter handle. The catheter runs parallel to the insertion tube of the endoscope. (*C*) OTSC device loaded onto clear plastic cap on tip of scope. (*Courtesy of* Aponos Medical, Kingston, NH, with permission.)

perforations (**Fig. 2**C, D). The key element to technical success is the positioning of the lesion within the OTSC cap. Misfiring to 1 side of a lesion can affect successful deployment of a second clip over the defect. Reloading a clip can be performed, if a second attempt is needed. More typically, suboptimal closures can be finished with supplemental mucosal clip placements.

OverStitch Endoscopic Suturing System

The OverStitch endoscopic suturing system is composed of an end cap, needle driver handle, and an anchor exchange catheter. The distal tip of the endoscope is attached to the end cap, which has a hinged, curved, hollow needle body, which opens and closes in an arc, simulating the curved needle used in surgery. The needle driver handle opens and closes the suture arm. The suture cassette contains a suture that is attached to a needle tissue anchor and attaches to the suture arm. After a stitch has been placed, the anchor exchange catheter allows the tip of the needle anchor to be exchanged, the needle body withdrawn from the tissue, leaving the stitch in place, and then reloaded with the needle for the next stitch.[3]

One advantage of this suturing method is versatility. The system allows continuous or interrupted stitches to be made of various lengths.[14,24] The endoscope does not need to be removed from the lumen for reloading needles or cinching. Furthermore, suturing is completed with the equivalent of intracorporeal knot tying, using a cinching device.[24] Location and depth of suture placement and needle penetration can be accurately identified.[13] Tissue depth, especially full thickness, is facilitated by use of a tissue screw catheter (Helix, Apollo Endosurgery, Austin TX), which is deployed through the second channel of the endoscope.

Cardiac Septal Defect Occluder

The ASO is a dumbbell-shaped device composed of 2 self-expandable, umbrella-shaped disks made of nitinol mesh with polyester fabric, which are constrained within a 70-cm delivery catheter and deployed over an endoscopically placed guidewire

(**Fig. 1**).[15,17] The occluder is an FDA-approved device for the closure of atrial septal defects.[15] The polyester fabric is sewn securely to each disk to help close the hole and serve as a foundation for growth of tissue over the occluder after placement.[16,17] The device also possesses radiopaque marker bands, which can be used under fluoroscopy.[17] Although the delivery catheter is too short to be passed through an endoscope, a guidewire can be inserted under endoscopic guidance. When the endoscope is withdrawn, the occluder can be introduced over the guidewire. The device apposes the wall on each side of the defect, thus occluding it and creating a platform for subsequent tissue ingrowth and epithelization.[17] These devices can be found in a variety of waist diameters and lengths, depending on the defect that needs closure.[3] Correct positioning of the device before deployment is critical for successful tissue apposition.

OUTCOMES
Over-the-Scope Clip

Overall success rates of OTSC in the literature range from 75% to 100% for closure of iatrogenic GI perforations, 38% to 100% for closure of GI fistulas, 50% to 100% for anastomotic leaks, and 71% to 100% for bleeding lesions.[11,12] The OTSC system has been used to repair perforations at esophageal, gastric, small bowel, and colonic sites.[25–27] Voermans and colleagues[25] reported successful endoscopic closures by location: 100% success for esophageal, 100% for gastric, 75% for small bowel, and 92% for colonic perforations.

Another study[28] examined the efficacy of the OTSC in the management of both acute and chronic colorectal postsurgical leaks and fistulas. The study included cases in which the fistula orifice was less than 15 mm in maximum diameter and no abscess or luminal narrowing was seen. In 14 consecutive patients, the overall success was 86% (7/8) in acute fistulas and 83% (5/6) in chronic fistulas. Two cases of rectovaginal fistulas were included in the study. Not only has the OTSC proved itself to be important in the management of acute and chronic GI closures, its use has been shown to decrease the need for surgery and length of hospital stay.[29]

OTSC has been used for expanding indications, including stent fixation. A recent retrospective case series by Mönkemüller and colleagues[10] evaluated outcomes of patients treated with the OTSC. Indications included GI bleeding, gastrocutaneous fistulas, esophagotracheal or esophagopleural fistula, resection of submucosal tumor, stent fixation, and anastomotic leak after esophagectomy. A total of 20 OTSC system applications were used in 16 patients with various GI defects, with an overall success rate of 75% (12 of 16 patients). The highest success rates were found in patients with GI bleeding (100%), whereas lower rates were found in patients with esophagotracheal or pleural fistulae (4 of 6 patients, 66%). These results were supported by data in a retrospective review by Baron and colleagues,[1] which found that in 45 patients treated with OTSC, immediate hemostasis was achieved in 100% of patients treated for GI bleeding and anastomotic leaks and fistulas were closed in 65% of patients.

Von Renteln and colleagues[8] compared standard TTS clips and OTSC for closure of NOTES gastrostomies in animals. This study found that OTSC in combination with a twin grasper was able to safely and efficiently close NOTES gastrostomies up to 18 mm in diameter and had a decreased risk of leakage and intra-abdominal infection when compared with closure with standard TTS clips.

The relatively recent evolution of this technology is accompanied by scant data regarding the long-term efficacy and potential adverse events of the OTSC. There are no current reports of adverse events arising in the GI tract secondary to clip placement.[11] Voermans and colleagues[25] found 19 of 24 clips to be present on follow-up endoscopy 6 months after OTSC placement for perforations of the GI tract.

OverStitch Endoscopic Suturing System

The first case reports of the endoscopic OverStitch device were for closure of a gastrocutaneous fistula that was refractory to closure with TTS clips and glue and direct closure of a persistent esophagopleural fistula for which a stent was also fixed by suture.[13,30] The suturing system has subsequently been used successfully to close a variety of lesions, including acute perforations, persistent gastrocutaneous fistulas, large mucosal defects, and full-thickness resection sites in both the stomach and colon.[13,14] It has also been used to fix esophageal stents in place and prevent migration and suture ulcers.[24] The use of endoscopic suturing to prevent spontaneous covered stent migration (see **Fig. 3**) has been valuable, because fully covered self-expandable metal stents are being used more frequently in the management of perforations and fistulas, but have high migration rates ($\leq$30%).[24,31]

A recent study[32] evaluated the use of the endoscopic suturing system for pouch and chiefly anastomosis revision in the Roux-en-Y gastric bypass patient with weight regain over time. Full-thickness tissue plications can be placed in the gastric pouch, providing volume reduction in those patients with an enlarged pouch. In most patients, the anastomosis can be reduced in size to 10 mm or less. The procedure was technically feasible, safe, and efficacious, with technical success achieved in 100% of patients.

A forerunner suturing system, the Eagle Claw VII, has been shown to be a feasible alternative for gastrostomy closure in animal models.[33] Although closure times with the Eagle Claw were longer than that of TTS clips, the endoluminal pneumatic bursting pressures for Eagle Claw VII were significantly higher than that of Endoclips.

Bursting pressure measurements with the OverStitch suturing system exceed those of the OTSC and compare with hand-sewn closures. The OverStitch endoscopic suturing system was determined to be a safe device for suturing in an in vivo human colon model in 4 patients undergoing elective colectomy.[34] The sutures were consistently placed at the proper depth, with no significant risks for iatrogenic injury.

Cardiac Septal Defect Occluder

Several case reports have been described regarding the use of cardiac septal defect occluders for the closure of GI fistulas and anastomotic dehiscence, with varying degrees of success.[15–18,35]

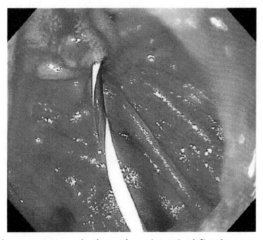

Fig. 4. Wire placed transcutaneously through an intestinal fistula.

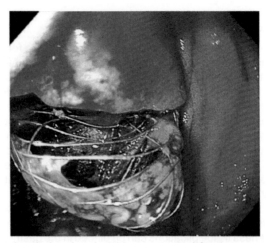

Fig. 5. Cardiac septal occluder placed within an intestinal fistula.

Two cases involving tracheoesophageal fistulas (TEF) had significantly different results. Coppola and colleagues[16] described the use of the ASO, which subsequently migrated into the bronchial tree and had to be removed from the middle lobe bronchus, placing the patient at risk for airway obstruction. Repici and colleagues[17] described the successful use of the ASO for a TEF. A gastrografin study immediately after deployment of the occluder showed fistula closure. Follow-up at 1, 3, and 8 months showed that the fistula remained closed and there was partial re-epithelialization of the mucosa covering the occluder.

One case report described the use of both the ASO and the CardioSEAL septal repair implant (NMT Medical, Boston, MA) in a patient with gastrocolonic fistula who was a poor surgical candidate. Multiple endoscopic attempts at fistula closure with TTS clip placement and biodegradable plug were unsuccessful.[15] A final attempt was made using the ASO and 3 mL cyanoacrylate glue to create a watertight seal. A gastrografin enema confirmed fistula closure, and the patient resumed enteral feeding 48 hours later. Four months later, the fistula was found to be patent. The CardioSEAL device was successfully deployed and once again used in conjunction with cyanoacrylate glue for closure. Four months later, the device was found to be in good position, but there was no evidence of epithelialization over the device membrane.

Data in animal models suggest that gastrostomy closure with cardiac septal occluders is efficacious and safe.[36] At follow-up endoscopy in the animal models, there were no signs of adhesions, peritonitis, or abscess formation.

We used the device to close an intestinal fistula via a transcutaneously placed occluder under direct endoscopic visualization (**Figs. 4** and **5**).

SUMMARY

Intraluminal devices are available to allow endoscopic closure of acute and chronic GI wall defects, including spontaneous and iatrogenic perforations, anastomotic leaks, and fistulas. As more experience is gained, these devices and methods will undoubtedly improve.

REFERENCES

1. Baron TH, Song LM, Ross A, et al. Use of an over-the-scope clipping device: multicenter retrospective results of the first US experience (with videos). Gastrointest Endosc 2012;76(1):202–8.

2. Binmoeller KF, Grimm H, Soehendra N. Endoscopic closure of a perforation using metallic clips after snare excision of a gastric leiomyoma. Gastrointest Endosc 1993;39(2):172–4.
3. ASGE Technology Committee, Banerjee S, Barth BA, et al. Endoscopic closure devices. Gastrointest Endosc 2012;76(2):244–51.
4. Seebach L, Bauerfeind P, Gubler C. "Sparing the surgeon": clinical experience with over-the-scope clips for gastrointestinal perforation. Endoscopy 2010; 42(12):1108–11.
5. Al Ghossaini N, Lucidarme D, Bulois P. Endoscopic treatment of iatrogenic gastrointestinal perforations: an overview. Dig Liver Dis 2014;46(3):195–203. http://dx.doi.org/10.1016/j.dld.2013.09.024.
6. Yoshikane H, Hidano H, Sakakibara A, et al. Endoscopic repair by clipping of iatrogenic colonic perforation. Gastrointest Endosc 1997;45(5):464–6.
7. Keller DS, Delaney CP. Current evidence in gastrointestinal surgery: natural orifice translumenal endoscopic surgery (NOTES). J Gastrointest Surg 2013; 17(10):1857–62.
8. Von Renteln D, Vassiliou MC, Rothstein RI. Randomized controlled trial comparing endoscopic clips and over-the-scope clips for closure of natural orifice transluminal endoscopic surgery gastrotomies. Endoscopy 2009;41(12):1056–61.
9. Zhang J, Samarasena JB, Milliken J, et al. Large esophageal fistula closure using an over-the-scope clip: two unique cases. Ann Thorac Surg 2013;96(6):2214–6.
10. Mönkemüller K, Peter S, Toshniwal J, et al. Multipurpose use of the "bear claw" (over-the-scope-clip system) to treat endoluminal gastrointestinal disorders. Dig Endosc 2014;26(3):350–7.
11. Singhal S, Changela K, Papafragkakis H, et al. Over the scope clip: technique and expanding clinical applications. J Clin Gastroenterol 2013;47(9):749–56.
12. Mennigen R, Colombo-Benkmann M, Senninger N, et al. Endoscopic closure of postoperative gastrointestinal leakages and fistulas with the over-the-scope clip (OTSC). J Gastrointest Surg 2013;17(6):1058–65.
13. Kantsevoy SV, Thuluvath PJ. Successful closure of a chronic refractory gastrocutaneous fistula with a new endoscopic suturing device (with video). Gastrointest Endosc 2012;75(3):688–90.
14. Kantsevoy S, Bitner M. Endoscopic suturing closure of large mucosal defects after endoscopic submucosal dissection is technically feasible, fast, and eliminates the need for hospitalization (with videos). Gastrointest Endosc 2014;79(3):503–7.
15. Melmed GY, Kar S, Geft I, et al. A new method for endoscopic closure of gastrocolonic fistula: novel application of a cardiac septal defect closure device (with video). Gastrointest Endosc 2009;70(3):542–5.
16. Coppola F, Boccuzzi G, Rossi G, et al. Cardiac septal umbrella for closure of a tracheoesophageal fistula. Endoscopy 2010;42(Suppl 2):E318–9.
17. Repici A, Presbitero P, Carlino A, et al. First human case of esophagus-tracheal fistula closure by using a cardiac septal occluder (with video). Gastrointest Endosc 2010;71(4):867–9.
18. Lee HJ, Jung ES, Park MS, et al. Closure of a gastrotracheal fistula using a cardiac septal occluder device. Endoscopy 2011;43(Suppl 2):E53–4.
19. Kouklakis G, Zezos P, Liratzopoulos N, et al. Billroth II gastrectomy complicated by gastrojejunocolonic fistulas, treated endoscopically with a cardiac septal defect closure device. Endoscopy 2010;42(Suppl 2):E134–5.
20. Moran E, Gostout C, McConico A, et al. Assessing the invasiveness of NOTES perforated viscus repair: a comparative study of NOTES and laparoscopy. Surg Endosc 2012;26(1):103–9.

21. Bingener J, Loomis EA, Gostout CJ, et al. Feasibility of NOTES omental plug repair of perforated peptic ulcers: results from a clinical pilot trial. Surg Endosc 2013;27(6):2201–8.

22. Cios TJ, Reavis KM, Renton DR, et al. Gastrotomy closure using bioabsorbable plugs in a canine model. Surg Endosc 2008;22(4):961–6.

23. Bonin EA, Bingener J, Rajan E, et al. Omentum patch substitute for facilitating endoscopic repair of GI perforations: an early laparoscopic pilot study with a foam matrix plug (with video). Gastrointest Endosc 2013;77(1):123–30.

24. Kantsevoy SV, Bitner M. Esophageal stent fixation with endoscopic suturing device (with video). Gastrointest Endosc 2012;76(6):1251–5.

25. Voermans RP, Le Moine O, von Renteln D, et al. Efficacy of endoscopic closure of acute perforations of the gastrointestinal tract. Clin Gastroenterol Hepatol 2012; 10(6):603–8.

26. Donatelli G, Vergeau BM, Dritsas S, et al. Closure with an over-the-scope clip allows therapeutic ERCP to be safely performed after acute duodenal perforation during diagnostic endoscopic ultrasound. Endoscopy 2013;45(Suppl 2):E392–3.

27. Mangiavillano B, Arena M, Masci E. Treatment of a sigmoid perforation with an over-the-scope clip during diagnostic colonoscopy. Clin Gastroenterol Hepatol 2014;12(6):xxi–xxii.

28. Arezzo A, Verra M, Reddavid R, et al. Efficacy of the over-the-scope clip (OTSC) for treatment of colorectal postsurgical leaks and fistulas. Surg Endosc 2012; 26(11):3330–3. http://dx.doi.org/10.1007/s00464-012-2340-2.

29. Gubler C, Bauerfeind P. Endoscopic closure of iatrogenic gastrointestinal tract perforations with the over-the-scope clip. Digestion 2012;85(4):302–7.

30. Bonin EA, Wong Kee Song LM, Gostout ZS, et al. Closure of a persistent esophagopleural fistula assisted by a novel endoscopic suturing system. Endoscopy 2012;44(Suppl 2 UCTN):E8–9.

31. Fujii LL, Bonin EA, Baron T, et al. Utility of an endoscopic suturing system for prevention of covered luminal stent migration in the upper GI tract. Gastrointest Endosc 2013;78(5):787–93.

32. Jirapinyo P, Slattery J, Ryan MB, et al. Evaluation of an endoscopic suturing device for transoral outlet reduction in patients with weight regain following Roux-en-Y gastric bypass. Endoscopy 2013;45(7):532–6.

33. Liu L, Chiu PW, Teoh AY, et al. Endoscopic suturing is superior to endoclips for closure of gastrotomy after natural orifices translumenal endoscopic surgery (NOTES): an ex vivo study. Surg Endosc 2014;28(4):1342–7. http://dx.doi.org/10.1007/s00464-013-3280-1.

34. Pauli EM, Delaney CP, Champagne B, et al. Safety and effectiveness of an endoscopic suturing device in a human colonic treat-and-resect model. Surg Innov 2013;20(6):594–9.

35. Cardoso E, Silva RA, Moreira-Dias L. Use of cardiac septal occluder device on upper GI anastomotic dehiscences: a new endoscopic approach (with video). Gastrointest Endosc 2012;76(6):1255–8.

36. Perretta S, Sereno S, Forgione A, et al. A new method to close the gastrotomy by using a cardiac septal occluder: long-term survival study in a porcine model. Gastrointest Endosc 2007;66(4):809–13.

Moving?

Make sure your subscription moves with you!

To notify us of your new address, find your **Clinics Account Number** (located on your mailing label above your name), and contact customer service at:

Email: journalscustomerservice-usa@elsevier.com

800-654-2452 (subscribers in the U.S. & Canada)
314-447-8871 (subscribers outside of the U.S. & Canada)

Fax number: 314-447-8029

Elsevier Health Sciences Division
Subscription Customer Service
3251 Riverport Lane
Maryland Heights, MO 63043

*To ensure uninterrupted delivery of your subscription, please notify us at least 4 weeks in advance of move.

Printed and bound by CPI Group (UK) Ltd, Croydon, CR0 4YY

03/10/2024

01040497-0016